ALMOST GONE

The Bay house before and after Hurricane Katrina

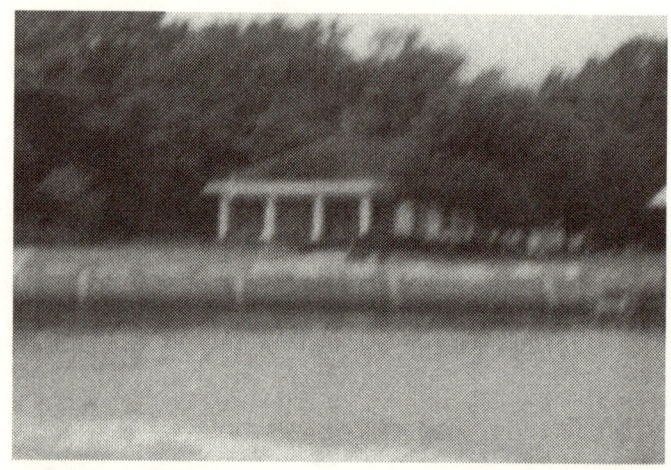

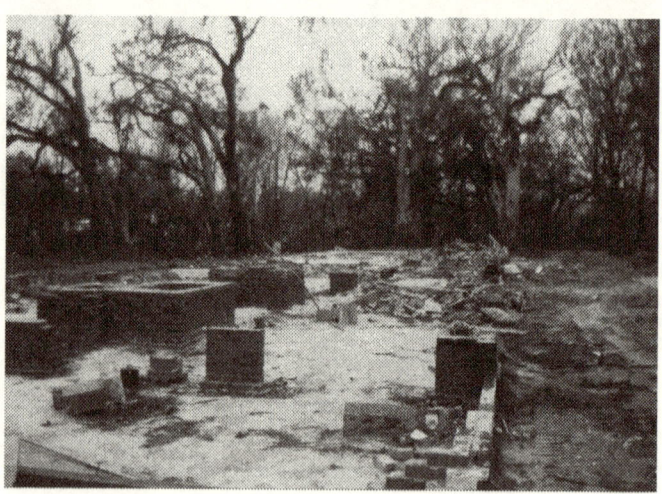

My first home in Waveland before and after Hurricane Katrina

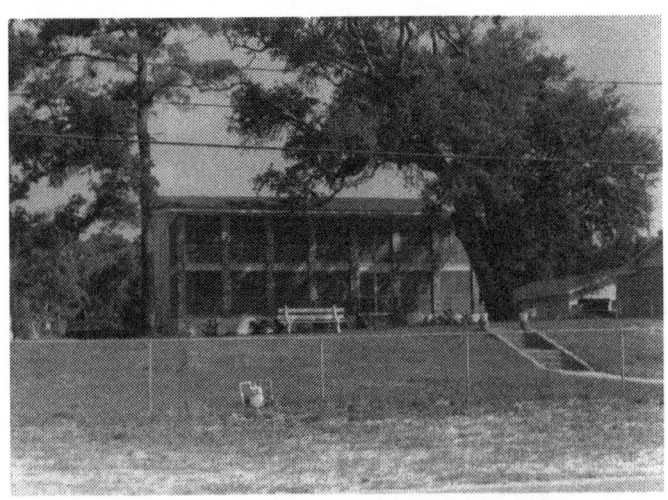

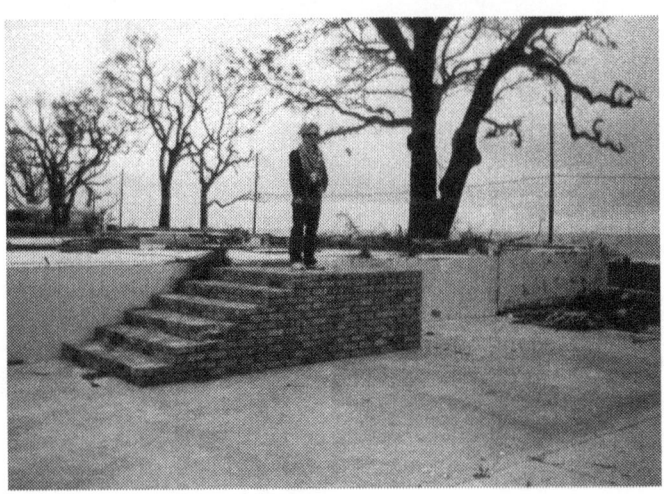

This image could also be: Gene's house, Aunt Peggy's house, Rosemary's house, the list goes on and on. They are all…almost gone…but not forgotten.

ALMOST GONE

Carol Taylor Lander

iUniverse, Inc.
New York Lincoln Shanghai

ALMOST GONE

iUniverse books may be ordered through booksellers or by contacting:

iUniverse
2021 Pine Lake Road, Suite 100
Lincoln, NE 68512
www.iuniverse.com
1-800-Authors (1-800-288-4677)

This is the true story of one woman's experiences with death, divorce, and cancer, then Katrina.

ISBN-13: 978-0-595-39156-1 (pbk)
ISBN-13: 978-0-595-83542-3 (ebk)
ISBN-10: 0-595-39156-7 (pbk)
ISBN-10: 0-595-83542-2 (ebk)

Printed in the United States of America

ALMOST GONE...

Almost gone...the carefree days of my youth.

Almost gone...the dreams of living happily ever after with my prince charming.

Almost gone...my roots.

Almost gone...my family.

Almost gone...my life.

Contents

Foreword

I started this book four years ago after my mother suddenly passed away from a brain tumor. I wrote my memoirs for many reasons, mostly for my own mental therapy.

As with so many of my projects, I was never quite able to finish the final details and set the ball in motion. Many people have read the incomplete version of this story and encouraged me to continue, but I was always stuck: stuck without an ending, and without a title. My dad, now eighty-five, really wants me to complete this, and after the past traumatic year, I think now is the time.

Now, where the book starts will be where the book ends. My beloved hometown, Bay St. Louis, Mississippi, is almost gone. Six months have passed since Hurricane Katrina, the largest national disaster in our country's history, devastated our Gulf Coast. I saw it six weeks after the storm and did not shed a tear. Shock, disbelief, and maintaining strength for the family and friends who lost everything did not allow me to express my feelings. It is only now, alone with my laptop, that I can look at the photographs of our homes in Bay St. Louis and feel so many emotions. I cry for all the wonderful times that we shared at those places. Oh, so many memories. Almost gone...but not forgotten.

Before I went to see the remains of our family home, my sister in-law Margaret took me to the area of the beach where my Aunt Dot lived. She had moved into her beachfront home fifty-one years ago as a bride, and she actually stayed in her home during Katrina! Her home had survived Hurricane Camille in 1969, the past benchmark of hurricanes, so, like many others, Aunt Dot and her brother decided to ride it out. By a miracle, they survived, but the house, which dated back to the 1840's, was severely damaged. I was shocked to see the skeletal remains. I remembered walking that same stretch of beach after Hurricane Camille, when the storm surge had come right up to Aunt Dot's front door. It looked like something took a huge bite out of the street, but saved her home.

This time, though, the wind and waves were too strong. Those special times at her home, eating cookies with her daughter, Noel, playing hide and seek in the maze of rooms, sneaking over to check on Great Aunt "Tonkeet" next door, sliding on large cardboard boxes down to the beach, all came rushing back to me. What wonderful times we had, and how thankful I am that our Aunt Dot survived. Almost gone…

As we drove through the back streets we passed our first home on Second Street. It was a long block away from the beach on high ground, and it had survived Hurricane Camille, so I was anxious to see how it fared. At first glance, it looked intact, and then I noticed the trailer sitting in the driveway. The wind and water had severely damaged the house, but it was repairable.

Our drive up to North Beach was heart wrenching. Beer in hand, I was preparing for a shock. What I saw was indescribable. The concrete Bay Bridge that had connected Bay St. Louis to Pass Christian was gone! This was no small road, but a main four-lane highway that was entirely washed away! Nothing but a few pilings remained. I remembered all the trips across that bridge to party as a teenager at Henderson Point and Bennie French's restaurant. So many years ago, so much fun.

Most recently, while driving that bridge at least twice a day while Dad was in Gulfport Memorial Hospital for his life saving bypass surgery just six weeks before Katrina, I had become very nostalgic. It was so beautiful, and I wondered wouldn't it be nice to have a place on the coast to share with my adult children and future grandchildren one day? To have them see and appreciate this beauty: the massive old oak trees that lined the streets, the sparkling Mississippi Sound with its shrimp boats and sea gulls and pelicans floating peacefully overhead, the elegant mansions built a century ago for prosperous New Orleanians escaping the city's heat. I remember talking to my sister-in-law in Michigan about this beautiful scenery as she called to inquire about my Dad and me during Hurricane Dennis. "Dear God, please spare this special area," I recall praying after hanging up from Ellen. My prayers were answered for Dennis, but not for Katrina.

Approaching North Beach Boulevard, flashbacks came to me. My sister, Sue, and I were walking after hurricane Camille, and saw nothing but brown, black, and trees with roots showing. Again, scenes from a war zone flooded my brain as I tried to stay in the present. Where are we? Where is the Lamb's house? Aunt Peggy's House? Basil's house? Was it not so long ago that we were here for his annual fourth of July party with Mom and Dad parading to the Yacht Club to hear the band Deacon John and the Ivories? Did that really happen in this desolate place or am I dreaming this? I wondered as we slowly eased along. Where was Polly's yellow cottage? Was it just weeks ago that I stayed there while Dad had his heart surgery? Did Aunt Peggy get her things out? Her beautiful antiques? Where is she now? All these questions racing in my mind as I try to absorb just a fraction of the emotions my friends and family must be feeling. There are no words to describe this kind of devastation.

We pass the harbor, and of course there is no yacht club. This will be the second or third time we have lost our favorite place for socializing. Our family has been a part of the Bay Waveland Yacht Club family for as long as I can remember and now the third generation has been enjoying the camaraderie and boating fun. No sunfishes, no flying scots, no ski boats, no fishing boats line the harbor. A few piling made it, that is all.

With no frame of reference, it is hard to determine where you are, and then you see it. A large piece of plywood was perched in the yard with black spray paint and the name Benvienutti. Our ever so fun loving neighbor Joe D marked his land with the sign, so I know we are next. I was told it was a good day to see the property, since the sky was blue. Now, I understand.

Truthfully, there is no good day to see this. Total devastation. A slab, uprooted trees with clothes flying like flags in the breeze. Pieces of wood, bricks, trash, kitchen utensils, furniture, shoes, stuff everywhere. A few steps later, more bricks, and I run into what once was our indoor pool. No more pool house. It now lies awkwardly between a dozen huge trees that have been up rooted.

We had over twenty years of fun in that pool. Mom swam laps almost daily, and I went into labor with Elizabeth while swimming in that pool. So many memories. Now, brown, black, and silence. Heart wrenching.

Then, there they are! Mardi Gras beads! And lots of them. Hanging from the trees, perched from limbs, stumps, and just lying on the ground. I tried to focus on these few bits of hope, and thus decided it was Mom's way of telling me to hold on. Hold on to the past, hold on to the memories, and hold on to the fun. Oh, how she loved her adopted city, New Orleans. That was my sign from Mom that day, those beads. I knew I had to do it, to hold on for Mom. Tears were not allowed; there were just too many things to do, and no time for emotional outbursts. I had to hold on...

Charles Swindoll, a minister in the Dallas area, writes about the importance of attitude. It has been my inspiration for so many years now, again I must remember "We cannot change the past or the inevitable." He says, "I am convinced that life is 10% what happens to me and 90% how I react to it".

I am reacting to this tragedy with sadness in so many ways. The loss of my childhood home, the town that helped raise me, my own first home in Waveland where my girls were born, and the past I will not be able to share with my children. But I am also, so thankful. So thankful that the lives of my father, my brothers and their families, my extended families and those wonderful people in the Bay-Waveland area were spared. These are the real heroes. These people who will never forget that horrible day, when they didn't know if they would live or die. These people who have the courage to persevere with the barest of necessities. These people who shared whatever they had to help their neighbor. Rich, poor, white, black, purple, no one escaped Katrina's wrath.

To these remarkably brave people, especially my brothers Dean and Gene and their families who now are picking up the pieces and building new lives, you are my heroes, and I dedicate this book to you.

I do believe life is fragile and everyday is a gift. Life is impacted by many factors, and everyone has a story. Mom always wanted to write a book about our family, we had so many great stories to tell. She never slowed down long enough to do it, so I did. It seems right to finish my story now.

Thanks and Acknowledgements

This has been a very long process, (I was a science major) and to my wonderful husband and very patient children I thank you. Now you know why your Mom is the way she is!!

To my sister Sue for always being there for me. To my sister Dianne for your wisdom and extreme patience in pulling me through English 101 at LSU, and for all the assistance in editing and encouragement you gave me to finish this. To Charlotte, for without her computer expertise this would never have made it to the publisher. To my incredibly talented and creative nephew Whitney for his time and energy developing the book cover I thank you so much. I am also deeply indebted to Blake, for pulling this all together and making it work. You are the best.

To my Dad, Potsy, for all you have done for me especially, that eternally optimistic attitude!

In memory of Bob and Margaret Lander for accepting me and for raising Bob to be such a special man.

Finally, to my Mom, my angel, the driving force behind this book, this is written in your memory.

The Taylor family moved to Bay St. Louis, Mississippi in 1953

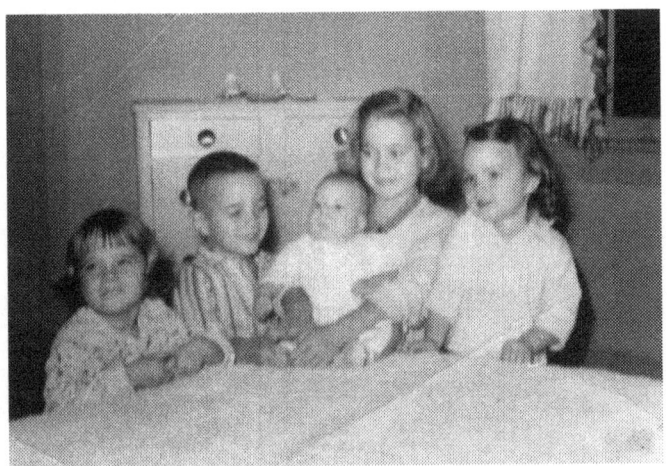

Sue, Dean, Dianne, baby Gene, and Carol

The five children in the back yard of our Second Street home in Bay St. Louis five years later.

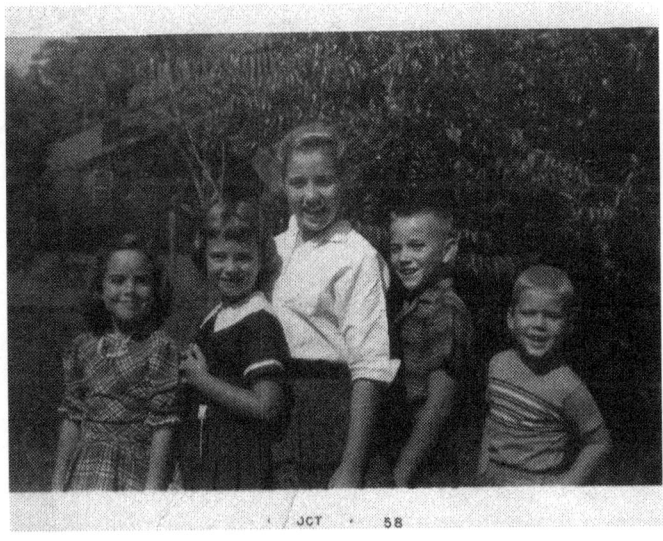

1

The Semi Southern Belle from Bay St. Louis

There are many different types of Southern Belles. Being born in New Orleans and growing up on the Mississippi Gulf Coast I've been around numerous varieties. The "true blooded" belles were of course from the "old money" families and had their name on the waiting list at Sacred Heart Academy before they were even born. These young women had ties to the gorgeous mansions on St. Charles Ave. and were the debutantes for the Rex, Comas, and Momus Krewes during the Mardi Gras season. That was just common knowledge in the Crescent City.

I knew having a mother that was a Yankee, and a father from Virginia or Maryland (where ever he chose to claim that day), that I would Never, Ever, be in the REAL clique, so I qualified for the Semi Belle. That was OK, for I enjoyed many of the benefits of the lifestyle without the responsibilities.

I enjoyed those wonderful years growing up in Bay St. Louis, Mississippi. Daddy was a salesman and left Mom home from Monday through Friday with 5 children under 7 to raise. Mom was a rock. As a Yankee, from Minnesota, Elizabeth, "Penny" found Dad when she took off to work in Panama during WW2. There she met the handsome Army Private, Taylor. They soon married, and when the war was over decided to settle in New Orleans with baby Dianne, since they both hated cold weather.

Dad's jobs eventually took us to "The Bay" a wonderful small town of 4,000 fine people and three or four knuckleheads. I kid you not! There was a sign as you entered the town of Bay St. Louis, Mississippi that read, "WELCOME TO BAY ST. LOUIS, HOME OF 3,999 FINE PEOPLE AND 3 OR 4 KNUCKLE HEADS." Well, they were not kidding!

This rural, "Mayberry type" town taught me the first of many life lessons.

Lesson 1: Accept all different kinds of people.

Take Bobo, the Hobo. Well, Bobo was probably the first homeless person I had ever noticed, but back then we didn't have homeless. Bobo was a small framed man that just stood on different corners of the town dressed in his white suit and waved to people saying "Hullo" all the time. Of course we were all scared of him. I'm not sure why, because he was not a scary kind of guy. As kids would do, we would dare each other to go up to speak to him.

Being the fourth child in the family, I was always looking to outdo the others, so of course I volunteered to go give BOBO a snow cone one day. As all the neighborhood kids watched, I ran up to him and handed him the snow cone and ran away as fast as my short, fat legs would take me. Of course he loved it, and said "Thank you" about a million times, but I was still running so I only heard the first one. After that, we all realized that he was not going to hurt anyone, he was just different, and from then on nobody was afraid of BOBO. We just accepted that he was indeed one of the towns "Knuckle Heads".

Then we had Mary Govan. Mary was an ancient, (probably in her forties) African-American woman who drove a truck around town and lived on a pig farm. This in itself was very strange since back then women NEVER drove trucks, not to mention she also smoked a PIPE as she was driving around delivering her pigs! Naturally she was a target. All the prank calls we kids could get away with were to Mary Govan's house, asking about her pigs and how much they cost, etc., etc. We would of course wait till the wee hours of the morning to make these calls and she would get so angry and cuss at us and swear she would find our Daddy and have us "whipped." We just loved it.

Then there was Clarence, lovingly called "Bottlehead". Clarence's Mom dressed in the old style. She wore the "home on the prairie" long dress with the big bonnet. Now this was in the mid fifties, and we had advanced somewhat from that look in Mississippi. She had Clarence in a wagon and pulled him around town till she died. Then Clarence took up a bike and rode the streets. I heard that the town took care of him and gave him odd jobs, but all I remember was people saying, "There goes Bottlehead". Of course, his head was unusually shaped, like a bottle, thus his nickname. I think he is still around, probably the last of the knuckleheads.

Growing up in coastal Mississippi was a treat. Bay St. Louis in the fifties was the kind of place where even hardware salesman with large families could afford to belong to the local yacht club. We swam nine months a year, played with the neighborhood kids, never wore shoes, and learned about life from each other. When I was six years old, Dad won a ski boat during a sales promotion. That boat was the magnet that drew our family and friends together for many years. Mom was a fabulous water skier (she slalomed on one ski till she was in her 70's!) and she and Dad literally taught just about every child in Bay St. Louis between the ages of six and twelve how to ski. It was great. The beginning of our family "playing together."

I watched my parents work hard at home and at work, and we all had so much fun when we played. That was the best lesson I ever learned.

Lesson 2: Work hard and play hard.

2

Change Is Inevitable, and Belles Don't Like It!

With every end there is a new beginning. We reluctantly ended our "wonder years" and moved to the big city with Dad's promotion to a better territory. My younger brother, Gene, was in the second grade when we moved to Baton Rouge, Louisiana, and he was by far the biggest rebel. He ranted and raved the whole three-hour drive to our new home, stating he did not want to move to the city and he would never wear shoes no matter what! But as does happen, we adapted, he wore shoes, and we tried to fit in. Fortunately, we were able to keep our house in the Bay and would return as often as possible on weekends.

Mom and Dad, both only children themselves, and both raised by single parents, always wanted a large happy family. I don't know how they did it, but by and large we all were pretty happy.

As we all grew, Mom and Dad were able to keep the family close, a task that to this day I admire and strive to achieve. We were all so different. Dianne, the oldest, is the brilliant one. She has a memory that is incredible, and she breezed through school and married a young attorney during college. She went on the TV show Jeopardy when she was twenty-one, a new mom and recent college graduate. She won five episodes, and the staff loved her. They had her husband and baby on camera the last day of taping. She won enough money for their first new car. We were all so proud of her. Later when they moved back to Baton Rouge, and I was at Louisiana State University, we used to barter. I would baby-sit, and they would help me with my English papers. It took me awhile, but I finally got the hang of it!

Dean, two years younger than Di, challenged the folks like all first sons do. I am not sure if Mom kicked him out of the house two or three times during those college years. (I have repeated that history and booted my precious Ed out once already. Of course, he schmoozed his way back in, just like Dean did.) Somehow, he always managed to get back in her good graces. Those boys could always work Mom!

Sweet Sue, a year and a half younger than Dean, loved everybody and would give the shirt off her back if someone needed it. When she was in the third grade we had just received new baby dolls for Christmas, and Sue gave her Tiny Tears to a little poor girl in her class at Our Lady of the Gulf school. She also persuaded me to do the same. I wasn't quite so eager to part with mine, and to this day I wish I had saved my Tiny Tears. Why did that little girl need two? Sue always had a way to get me to go along with her way, mostly with guilt trips. My sister Dianne reminded me that Sue also gave away our treasured Madam Alexander dolls. Mom was both proud and furious and so was Di!

Being thirteen months younger than Sue and the baby girl, I was always trying to get attention. I guess that's why I was nicknamed "crazy Carol".

Gene, the baby, was two years younger than me. We started playing together in those early years at the Bay and carried it over through the years, with the help of our boat and our Bay house.

Mom got a little worried that Sue and I were not getting all the "proper training" we needed to be "ladies". In the fifth grade, when both Sue and I showed up with a D in conduct on our report card from playing with the boys at the local school, she panicked. The fact that we were Brownie dropouts didn't help us much either. So, Mom took action.

Sue, being the favorite, was enrolled in a Speed Reading class, and I was directed to Charm School! Charm School? Was this a joke? What had I done to deserve this? OK, I played sports with the boys, and I played basketball, but God forbid. Charm School? I was mortified. And bitter. They could send me to charm school but by God, I still did not HAVE to wear shoes nor did I have to be nice to other girls. Or act like a girl!

Six weeks later, Charm School graduation day, Mom came into my room and inquired as to what in the world I was doing with the "No Bugs Milady" shelf lining paper. I explained that at Charm School they told us that all ladies covered their shoeboxes with paper, and this was all I could find. She was laughing so hard and shaking her head. "All that money spent, and all she got from six weeks of training was for her to wrap her shoeboxes in NO BUGS MILADY?" She was sure I was hopeless. Guess I failed Charm School.

Dad had some insight that staying home with five kids was not an easy thing. So, fortunately, no matter how poor we were, he always agreed to have some kind of household help. Not maids. We loved those women, and they were definitely more like family. Mom taught us that. Treat everyone like they are family. We all bonded well, even with the worst of jobs.

Like the time Mom tried to get us to eat liver. Now ours was a serious casserole family since money was tight, and where she got this brainstorm I will never know! Dad did like the awful stuff. Being the depression child he was he liked all that junk (including Spam). So Mom slaves over the hot stove whipping up all this liver. The smell of the onions cooking was pretty tempting so we all sat in our designated seats on the long wooden benches which lined the kitchen table made from a hollow-core door, and proceeded to feast on what we thought would be a real delicacy. Dean took the first bite.

The chewing slowed to a mere chomp, and he was up and running. I took the next bite and within seconds began to hurl. Sue looked at my greenish color face then at the regurgitated liver on the floor, and her hand quickly hit her mouth. Too late. She couldn't hold it in, and the chain reaction continued. More vomit. By this time Mom had had enough. The foul smell on that black and white linoleum floor permeated through the house and she took off to hide and cry somewhere. Nobody was left but Albertine.

Albertine took one look at the mess and said, "I'm not cleaning that up." So, under Dianne's direction, we kids grabbed paper towels and started skating over the slimy floor. Each handful scooped up resulted in another round of hurling. It was a real barfarama.

Mom tried so hard to do everything, but often times she would need another pair of hands. Mornings before school were always tough. When we were in grammar school in the Bay especially, Mom could never quite get things together before we left for school, and many times she needed to bring our lunches to us later in the morning.

We were all so embarrassed. Poor Mom, she would either drive that old black 1948 Frazier, if it ran, or she would ride her bike to bring the sandwiches. (Too frequently, she rode the bike). She would cruise the playground till she found us and then proceed to yell, "Carol, Carol. I've got your bologna sandwich!" I would die a thousand deaths before I finally could make my way over and retrieve my sandwich. Day after day, bologna sandwiches. I was told how thankful I should be to have a sandwich considering all the starving children in the world. I thought a lot about all the starving children in China and just wished I could figure out a way to send those darn sandwiches over there!

Fortunately, all my friends knew that I hated bologna sandwiches, and they were willing to trade with me for just about anything on a daily basis. Thank goodness for friends!

Lesson 3: Mothers sometimes DO embarrass their children, and kids need to learn to get over it!

3

Belles Should Be Involved.

Down South, like most areas of the U.S., boys learn about involvement through sports activities. We start them young down here, and our favorite sport is football.

For the good southern belle, your first experience in group activities is in cheerleading. All belles have at some point in their lives been a cheerleader, and Sue and I began this journey at the tender ages of five and six.

The Brothers of Sacred Heart ran a day school and boarding school for "bad boys" as well as the Bay St. Louis locals, St. Stanislaus College. The annual Fleas vs. Flies game was the football Super Bowl for the school. No kidding, two "peewee" teams with little boys in the first grade, called fleas and flies! No parents in their right minds today would allow their precious babies anywhere close to a football field at that age, much less, suit them up to play!

Anyway, they did have cheerleaders (we know how important they are) and one day, Sue decided we should try out. She dragged me up to speak to the head Brother. We walked the mile, (it seemed like a mile), along the beach to the school, and begged to be cheerleaders. We were five and six years old! This was quite traumatic as I recall. I was scared to death of the big man in the long black robe. We walked in together holding hands looking like little Darla and one of her friends from the *Little Rascals* movie. Sue did all the talking and at age six she was able to "work her show" as well as she could at 26! Well, she was chosen, and I was told I was too young. The first of many rejections!

Cheerleading is serious business for "Belles" down South, and as you can see, we start young. This was the first of many sibling rivalries between Sue and me. Later in Baton Rouge, we both tried out for cheerleader. Fortunately for us, the good nuns somehow forgot about that vital aspect of sports, so we proceeded to organize the group and we chose ourselves to lead it!

Our cheerleading career was in full swing and we were on the road to being real Southern Belles. I never realized how far that cheerleading experience would take me, not until much later. I realize that I have tapped into that cheerleading mode every day at work for the past thirty years. A huge part of my job is motivating my patients to work hard and cheering for them as they succeed. Actually, that is my favorite part of my work, not just teaching them what to do, but also encouraging them to achieve their goals. Who said cheerleading was worthless?

Lesson 4: Get with the sports program but forget "real men's" work. Holding up the family is hard enough!

Mom pretty much did everything, but there were a few tasks she always refused to perform: pay bills, take out the trash, or fix things. Ladies just did not do such things.

While we lived in Baton Rouge, Dad would be out of town for extended periods, and Mom would "lose it" on a regular basis. Taking care of five kids and a house, dealing with raging menopausal hormones, and trying to quit smoking to boot, was just overwhelming…especially when you didn't pay the bills.

Frequently, we would have our power turned off. Mom just could not understand how that could happen. One time that happened, Dad was gone and the car was broken. When we came home from school Mom was crying and carrying on, until finally Daisy Mae, our wonderful house helper, decided she needed to take charge.

She settled Mom down and had her write the check. Sue and I jumped in Daisy's car and she drove like a "bat out of hell," weaving in and out of traffic in her big old Chevrolet, in rush hour traffic, trying to get to the electric company before it closed. We barely made it, and from then on Daisy became our hero. (She was already our best friend). When it was time to move with Dad's next promotion, we all tried to persuade Daisy to come with us, but she could not leave her "nest". We loved Daisy so much. She had truly become part of our family, and we would miss her terribly. She taught us to "take charge" when Mom got overwhelmed.

Mom always got stuck holding up the family. For every crisis we had, and we had many, Mom was our Savior. Not just for little traumas, but for big ones.

Take the time our friends from Michigan came to visit. The Foley family lived in the Bay when we did, but then moved back to Yankee land after a few years. They had two kids at the time, Missy and Tom. Tom, who was about two years old, happened to have the chicken pox when they came to visit.

As usual, Dad was out of town. After dinner one night, as Sue and I were headed for bed, we realized that the next day was a first Friday. This only sends chills down your spine if you attend a parochial school, and your special outfit for First Friday is dirty, and it is too late to get Mom to clean it without serious yelling.

So, we took matters into our own hands. White skirts were hand washed, and placed on sister Di's vertical radiator to dry. Mission accomplished. We headed to bed pleased we had averted another punishment.

Later that night, as fate would have it, the weather turned colder and the radiator stayed on for a prolonged period of time. You guessed it; we awoke to a faint scream of "OH, OH".

Mothers never really sleep (as long as kids are home) and within seconds, Mom had darted up the steps, and began beating the fire with a towel. Di was sent downstairs to call for help and the commotion began. Now just imagine an old upstairs with six sleeping children and two adults and one staircase. This could have really been disastrous! So, the fireman finally come and one takes a look at baby Tommy and asks, "What's the matter with him?" We nonchalantly say that he has the chicken pox, and panic erupts a second time. Seems there were some firemen that had never had "the pox" and they were spooked. No one seemed to get too close to the baby needless to say; they did their job and were out in a flash. Grown men afraid of the chicken pox…later I found out why they ran so fast!

Mom was such a pillar of strength for the "serious crisis" but then the hormones of menopause would surge, and she would be a mess for the mini crisis. It didn't help that she quit smoking during this life transition, so occasionally out of the blue, a major meltdown. Usually, of course, the frustration of being home alone with teenage kids was a pretty good precursor for one of her spells!

Take the time we were having dinner one night. Mom was a firm believer of family dinner times together. No matter how late our activities were scheduled, we always ate together. (I have repeated this with my own family). When the girls were finished getting everything ready, (yes we were sexist back then, the girls had "woman's work," and the boys had generally just trash duty!) we called the boys.

We waited for them to come in from playing outside, called, waited, called them again, waited, called again, til finally they arrived. Invariably we always had cold food. (One of my hang-ups to this day, I hate cold food). Then after a quick glance at the entrée, the looks began. One brother looked at the other, sister looked at brother, sister to sister, and spontaneously it began. The "Same old Slop" tune. Yep, we had our own rendition of "Three Blind Mice". We took the tune and replaced the words with "Same old Slop". As we beat our fists against the table we entered into our song, "Same old Slop, Same old Slop, That's all we got that's all we got. We have it every Monday night, Tuesday night, Wednesday night, when do we ever get anything right, just same old slop!"

Kids can be so cruel! That was the catalyst for a major melt down. Mom stood up from her seat at the head of the table, picked up her plate full of food, raised it high into the air and suddenly proceeded to throw it as hard as she could on the floor. It fell with a loud crash, and then we heard footsteps and a heavy door slam. Whoops! All five kids looked at each other with shocked expressions. Great. Now look what we have done! Then, we all started laughing. We couldn't stop…hum…what to do now?

When the severity of the situation finally sunk in we looked to our only hope, the baby, Gene. "Oh, no, not me. I'm not going in there! Why do you always send me to do the dirty work? Not me, not this time." He pleaded. We finally convinced him to just quietly sneak in her bedroom with a very remorseful expression, and bring her a new plate of food. (This time we put it on a plastic plate!) Poor Mom. We gave her such grief! He fulfilled his mission, but I'm not sure she ever ate that night.

Probably the highlight of Mom's life back then was when Dean would bring his friends home. She loved those teenage boys! He had a group of four or five regulars that landed at our house every afternoon after school for a quick cake or ice cream snack. They adored her since she was the "food mom". (Mom made a cake everyday back then.)

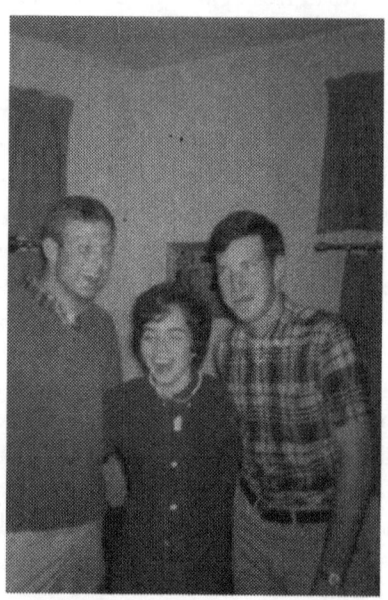

Dean's friends, Mickey and our beloved Don having fun with me in the Bay

Those guys were so funny. We would hear the escapades of their date life, and other adventures. Sue and I were particularly pleased because on a rare occasion they even included us! Our family would bring them to the Bay on weekends and we would all swim and ski all day. They were like big brothers to us, and we loved it.

I still remember the most embarrassing moment with those guys. We were all sitting in the back room on the bed and the guys start talking about sex. (Just out of the blue this subject came up!) Well, we were just old enough to know about "IT" but not really. So they decided it was time we learned the "fine points". Sue and I were so mesmerized when they started demonstrating the French kiss on a glass, we giggled and turned red, and did the old "you gotta be kidding" stuff, but as things progressed, we both pulled the blanket over our heads. We couldn't stand it any longer. We were so embarrassed, and we couldn't let them see our faces so we pulled the cover up over our heads! We were horrified, (they loved it) but we were determined to get through the entire session. Thankfully, they were only 16 and 17, and it was a short lesson!

We had good times during those years we went to the Bay for the summers. We would get together with our friends, sleep over at Polly's house and go to the beach. Brownish-green water and off white beach, it was after all a beach! I had been going to the infamous Bay Waveland Yacht Club and swimming and sailing the days away for years. One of our friends always had a little sunfish sailboat and we would pack it with soft drinks and our favorite snacks and head out across the Bay to the secluded area in Pass Christian. This was so fun, lying in the sun feeling the cool water running through your fingers as the boat heeled, and we glided through the waves. All day long we would talk teenage talk about boys, laugh and eat junk food! Little did we know that "the way we were" would catch up with us, and that we would pay the price for those many hours in the sun. We didn't need baby oil to get tan, because we were already tanned! The sun god just did his thing. Now at mid life we are all cursed by the scars of the "Sun Devil".

Summer days in the sun and nights on the beach. I remember my first beach party. We were at the Eagan's beach right down from the Yacht Club on North Beach Blvd. The "big kids" (our older siblings) were really having the party, we just happened to go too. The stacks of wood were piled high in an inverted V fashion, and at just the right moment it was lit. The fire lit up the sky, the stars were shining, and the waves crashed into the shore. A perfect night.

All the teens were there roasting marshmallows, and talking, and out of nowhere comes my "crush". Donald was one of seven or eight kids, and since his brothers were there he was allowed to go too. (That was the rationale for me too). Out of nowhere, he asked me if I wanted to walk to the Frostop and get a coke. I froze. Walk, alone in the dark, along the beach, under the Bay Bridge to get a coke? I was only in the 5th grade! But, what the heck, why not, and walk we did. I was so afraid to go under the Bay Bridge. It was so dark, and I am deathly afraid of all critters, rats, and snakes at the top of the list. I ran so fast and finally emerged to the starlight and that beautiful view of the giant root beer on top of the Frostop. Winded, an ready to sit a minute, Donald so gallantly asked me "What do you want,…for a nickel?" I paused a moment and replied, "A cherry coke." We drank our cokes and went back to the party. I was feeling quite smug when I met up with my siblings, until they found out that Donald gave me a nickel limit. "What do you want for a nickel?" Laugh, laugh, I heard about that for years, believe me. Older siblings can be such a pain!!

The good old days were so great. Not a care in the world. So many great memories.

4

The Scarlet Years: Trix and Legs in the Big Easy

All Southern belles hate change. And here we go again. The family now moved to the real big city. Dianne, the oldest was married. Dean was in college at Tulane University and the three youngest kids now moved to "the New Orleans Catholic private school scene," otherwise interpreted as all girls' and all boys' schools. Sue, Gene and I tried to make some sense out of this, but to no avail.

Gene survived by meeting a fabulous group of friends. Sue and I decide to eat ourselves sick. We missed our friends, and Mom and Dad were helpless. We ate pies and cried for six months til, finally, my brother Dean, saved us.

As a fraternity boy now, he thought it would be a great way for his two sisters to meet people by being Rush Girls at Tulane. Mom of course, was totally naïve to the ways of the fraternity world. She loved this idea because now Dean would be around to watch over us. Ha! What a joke!

We thanked God for opening our little window! Our junior and senior years in high school were taking on a new dimension. Goodbye high school boys, hello cute frat boys!

Needless to say, we had a ball. At 16 and 17 we were partying with the college boys every Friday and Saturday nights. We practiced all the Scarlet O'Hara moves and just waited for our "Rhett Butler" to ride up on his horse. We even got to dress like her if you were lucky enough to be invited to the KA "Old South" party. Sue went numerous times and I just fantasized about my turn. Of course, it never happened, but that was OK. I lived my turn through her. We were best friends and shared everything. Those were good times. Things were different back then. No crime, no drugs, drinking was the worst offense, but we had been prepared.

With Dad's new position, Mom had to assume the role of Southern Belle hostess. She was brilliant. Beautiful, gracious, and ever so semi southern she wooed all the top dogs of those big companies. We had parties for all occasions, especially around football season and the holidays. Mom always made all the food herself and fortunately for Sue and I, taught us to help. We would have 50–100 people over on a moments notice and pull it off better than any caterer ever could.

Dad's job was to teach us how to drink. He felt like if we were prepared to handle drinking, then we were less likely to get into trouble. (You know what I mean "trouble".) The drinking age in Louisiana, back then, was 18, and Dad didn't have a problem with that. He always said "If you can fight for your country at 18 you sure should be able to have a drink at 18". Thus our introduction to drinking started at 17.

Of course with Mardi Gras and all the other celebrations in New Orleans it is easy to start before that. There is always a party. Just look at the funerals. We have bands and people march! We live to party in the Big Easy! So by 16 you have spit out your first bourbon and coke, by 17 Dad is fixing them at home (so we can pass out without notice) and by 18 we are veterans. We out lasted so many frat boys it became a joke when we met with Dean at his frat house and asked for a lift home. He would just shake his head and say "another rookie" poor guy.

Lesson 5: Be Prepared

We rarely got in trouble back in those days, but one night we came real close. Two of our very close friends were also invited to the fraternity parties that weekend and we all decided to stay at our house. We had a great time getting ready trading clothes, makeup and all of that fun stuff. Even though we were not all going to the same frat house, they were down the street from each other so we were sure to meet up at some point.

Mom, in her loving way, loaded us up with spaghetti. No going out on an empty stomach ever at our house. So off we went for a fun evening. The night progressed in the usual fashion, drinking, dancing, more drinking, and more dancing. Then, the tidal wave hit. Out of nowhere came that wave of nausea. The room began to spin and I head for the bathroom. That in it's self was a fate worse than death at a frat house. But, I was desperate and I charged into the restroom and began to be sick. Oh yuck, spaghetti everywhere! Sue saw me sprint off the dance floor and followed just in time to hold my long hair away from my face as I proceeded to call "Ralph". "Why did Mom give us spaghetti?" was all she could say. "My new dress! OH, No not my new dress ruined!" I was devastated. I loved that dress and here I'd ruined it the very first night I wore it! I was so mad at myself! Another dating tip to remember...NEVER eat spaghetti before going out to a party!

As the party wound down we started toward the other frat house to see our friends. (Guess we all lost the dates somewhere along the line, the story of our date lives) The rain had begun, but we didn't care, it was still warm out. Then Sue noticed it. Her dress began to "draw up." "Carol, is this dress shrinking or am I just imagining it?" This was real. Another catastrophe. Her dress was not her dress at all, but our friend's NEW crepe dress. Now how were we supposed to know that crepe SHRINKS when it gets wet? I had no schooling in textiles at Charm School, and we were never able to afford a crepe dress in the past, so we were innocent by reason of ignorance!

So Sue proceeded to tug and pull on her dress (all in vain) as we walked down the street and we met up with our friend. "What happened to you?" I asked Polly. "I fell in a puddle and got mud all over the dress!" Three up, three down. All three dresses "gone with the wind". We were in for it, but we would "think about that tomorrow!"

Tomorrow came too soon. Mom entered our room around noon to wake us up, (not quite like Aunt Peggy used to with orange juice on a tray singing "Good morning girls, it's a bright new day never been used") and was appalled by the mess and the smell. Three dresses destroyed, thrown all over the floor. As she gingerly picked each one up, she asked, "What happened?" Our heads were pounding, and our eyes too heavy to open, so we pleaded for mercy. "Mom can we talk about this later? We are not ready to get up yet."

"Carol, that is your new dress. Oh, my it stinks sooo bad, what did you do?" "Later, Mom". In frustration, she marched toward big brother's room.

She then glanced out of his window and noticed that the family car was gone. "Dean, where is the car?" No answer. "Dean, Dean where is MY car?" "I don't know, Mom, it's on campus somewhere" and he rolled over. She bolted down the stairs screamming "Gar ree! Come help me! What am I going to do with these teenagers? Please!"

Mom somehow survived life with three teenage kids in the Big Easy, but it certainly was ANYTHING but EASY!

5

Southern Belles and Steel Magnolias

As Forrest Gump said, "Life is like a box of chocolates. You never know what you are going to get."

Our life during those college years was fun too. We made friends at school, had a good education, respected and even had fun with our parents. Then it hit. The Viet Nam war hit too close to home. Dean's best friend, Don, flunked out of LSU and was drafted. Our world was shattered. Don was not only like a member of the family, but my first secret love. When I needed a date to the Prom I asked Don. Sorority formal time, I took Don. He never new I was smitten for him, cause I was just "Dean's little sister". But the day he called and told us he had been drafted, we all prayed and cried.

Don seemed to have that sense too that this was it. He partied and played like there was no tomorrow, and when we all were saying our goodbyes at the airport, we all cried so hard. His biological family, and his adopted family. Nobody can explain that horrible fear/pain combination of sending a loved one to war. Thank God, that was the only time I ever had to do that.

Our fun life would never be the same. I cry as I think about how full of life he was and how he always made us laugh. And how my first love was so sweet to me, even when to him I was only "a little sister". Don survived a year and a half in Viet Nam. He wrote all of us letters, keeping the real details from Sue and me. I saved two of his letters, and just re-read them again the other day. The first letter was written when he was in basic training. He sounded so cocky. I knew he was still thinking this was a big joke by the stories he told. The second letter was quite a bit different. He was in the heart of the battle area, and was anything but cocky. He said he had stopped volunteering for the lead position, but somehow the Sergeant continued to assign him that post. (I am sure he was very good at his job that is why he kept getting picked for the position.) He wrote about how lucky he had been and hoped the "Big Man" would keep watching out for him. That was my last letter. It concluded with "See you in 264 days. Love, Don". Nine months is a long time.

Then one day, again leading the unit, he went ahead of his team into the jungle and it happened. He stepped on a land mine. Explosion. Gone. In an instant, such a young, wonderful young man was lost. I don't think our family ever really recovered from that first experience with losing a loved one. We were all so close, and this was not supposed to happen to us. But it did. Life is so fragile.

I don't think my brother Dean ever recovered. Over night, he grew old, and bitter, and then sad. He is much quieter now, and much more serious. In a flash, his youth was stolen. Or maybe it is growing up before your time. Whatever it was, it was my first real reality check, and I didn't like it at all. We all learned another lesson that day: Life is fragile and can be very short. In 2002, 32 years after we lost Don, we lost Mom quite suddenly. Dean said to us, "Now Mom is with Don."

Over time, our pain eased, but we never forgot about Don. I touched his name on the Viet Nam Memorial in Washington D.C. a few years ago, and relived so many of our wonderful times together. His fun loving spirit will always be with our family.

Lesson 6: Enjoy your Kids

We had forgotten about play for a while and now we needed it desperately. Mom knew. So she encouraged us on. We had Mardi Gras with all our friends. Actually, so many friends, we weren't sure who was friend and who was foe.

Some of my fondest memories were of those years in New Orleans. Mom and Dad were saints. As a parent now of three teenagers, I am amazed they held up so well. But, as we know, things were different back then.

Mom worried about so many things, but not about our friends or our time going out. Since they had been feeding our friends since high school, and partying with them in college, they felt pretty good with our choices. But the things they went through.

Like the time we had so many kids staying with us during Mardi Gras. Three kids in college and you get lots of company in New Orleans during this time. We had so many, this time that Mom, organized as she was, decided that after she fed us, (she always fed us) she would make a list of everyone's name and put it on the back door so that when we got in, the last person would lock the door. Great idea…in theory.

Now this house was better known as "The Castle" since it really looked like a castle. We bought it after Dad's latest promotion, from Old Lady Qualey who was using it as a boarding house for Tulane boys. Mom loved that old house and had worked her magic for about a year turning it into a not just a mansion, but, a family mansion. Thus its nickname, the Castle.

The Castle had three floors and a basement. Yep, in the city that is below sea level we did indeed have a basement. So we had lots of hiding areas. It also had a fire escape. We loved the fire escape. Jumping up and hauling those heavy metal steps down when you were drunk was just exhilarating. We would tiptoe past Mom and Dad's bedroom feeling so smug, then literally, fall head first, from the third floor window to the floor. Lots of times I forgot my keys on purpose just so I could use the fire escape. Oh Happy days!

That year at Mardi Gras, we had at least 15 partying college kids staying with us. That in itself is a disastrous combination, and add Mardi Gras celebration to this amalgam and it was non-stop commotion.

The first "drunk kid" to arrive home, bypassed the list and locked the door. Soon, all hell broke loose. We had kids climbing up the fire escape and banging on the doors at all hours of the night, not to mention those MIA's (missing in action).

The next morning, Mom checked the list and found obscenities written all over it. She found all of us alive and well (sort of) and decided to just go with the flow. Somehow, nothing serious ever happened back then. She trusted us completely. I learned how to trust from my Mom.

Sue and I, the almost twins, pretty much always shared the same friends. In high school, college and when I was in the Physical Therapy program at LSU we would get together for all the partying occasions.

Mom loved being the "adopted Medical School Mom". During the few breaks in the year when we had time off, the Med school boys always came over to our house. The food was good, the price was right and Mom and Dad graciously served you all you could endure. My two favorite memories of those years are classic stories.

In my first year at the Medical school (the physical therapy program was so new they didn't know where to put us so we were grouped with the medical school) I lived at home. Not only was it cheaper, but more conducive to studying. With Dean in the Navy and Sue and Gene at LSU in Baton Rouge, it was just Mom, Dad, Nana, and me. When LSU had a slow weekend Sue would come home to visit. We were the "dream team" of blind dates. Two cute girls in the same house! So, we accepted any and all blind dates, knowing that someday our "prince" would be one of these guys. Somehow though, all we ever seem to get were the "frogs".

When the "frogs" were really bad, one sure way to be rid of them forever was to take them up to the "cadaver lab" at the Med school. Sue had heard so much about my cadaver, Big Bertha, and she just had to see for herself. So one night at about 2 am, we snuck through the back entrance and up to the lab. We were petrified! Dark, eerie halls with skeletons hanging around everywhere and we just knew there had to be rats all over. But, we forged ahead, until we finally saw the big double doors. We opened the doors and low and behold, there were at least thirty med students in there! All dressed in there dissecting gear, eating candy bars, and drinking cokes! Sue was flabbergasted! She had NEVER seen anybody studying at two in the morning. The dates were appalled. First, the smell of embalming fluid is enough to knock you out, then to see cut up dead bodies and people actually eating around them is enough to make you hurl. They didn't stay long.

After the shock wore off, she realized what an opportunity this was! Like all good Southern belles, we never miss an opportunity to flirt, and here we were totally out numbered! I thought Sue was going to "toss her cookies" when they were showing off all the body parts, but, she held up good. Fainting would have been the appropriate response, but she wouldn't dare miss an opportunity to use her charm with so many cute guys around! The dates helped me hoist up Big Bertha, and when they saw her toe tag, and got a good whiff of her, they decided that was close enough. It goes without saying that the dates were indeed horrified and we never heard from them again. Two more names added to the "bastard tree". (Sue's secret diary of frogs).

As you have surmised by now, Sue and I did not have serious relationship experiences back in our college days. To this, little brother, Gene so lovingly nicknamed us "Mamie and Irma" in reference to the two "old maids" that resided down the street in Bay St. Louis, the Hale sisters.

However, Gene had learned flexibility. When his friends wanted to go out, and they could not find any other girls to go with them, our names were changed to Trix and Legs (two good barmaids names) and we stepped up. Southern belles and their nicknames. Thank God, I never got the "Bunny" "Peachie" or "Muffi" names!

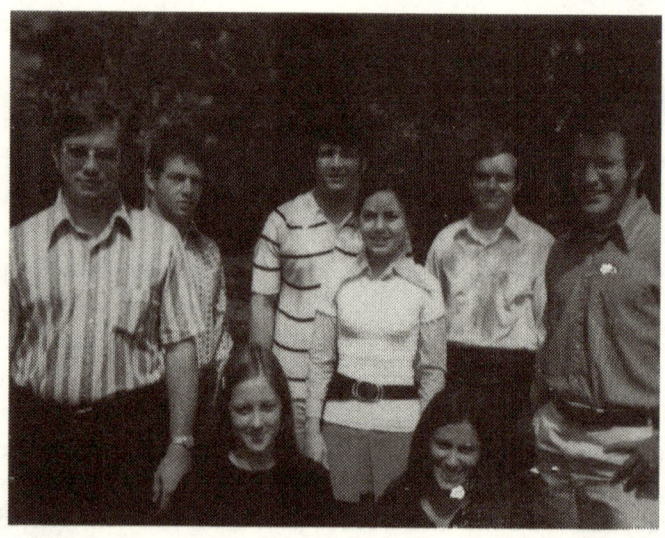

The Med school boys with the Physical Therapy girls on a weekend getaway to the Bay 1972
Jay, Bob, Lynn, Charlie, Mike, Wilda, Maureen and me

Charlie, Lynn, me
and Bob in the Bay

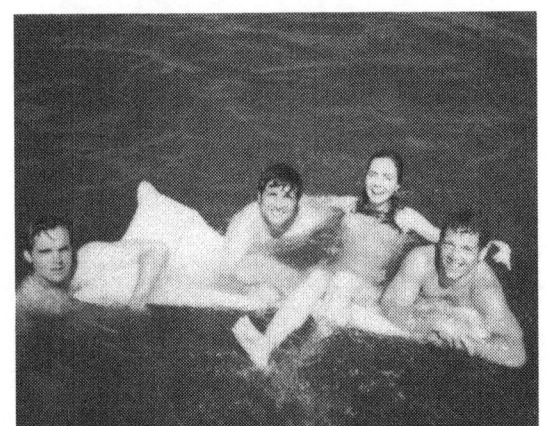

6

Fun Times

The highlight of my college days was the weekend Dad had convinced my four med school buddies to come paint our house in the Bay on their weekend off. The deal was this: we paint all day Saturday, go out on the boat Sunday, and you can eat and drink all you want. Those poor freshmen jumped on that deal so fast. And did we have fun!

The weekend started Friday afternoon leaving New Orleans after classes. Halfway there, we stopped at the White Kitchen restaurant lounge for a quick "toddie". Before I new it Mom had Jay Busby, (a fabulous dancer) on the dance floor and the party began. We eventually made it to the Bay, and with a quick change we were off to the Yacht Club for dinner. Now, this is not exactly a fancy establishment like many others on the Coast, but it was still THE PLACE to be seen on Friday nights.

My moment had finally arrived. Mom and Dad walked in, got the place buzzing, and then SILENCE. I walked in with my best Scarlet O'Hara grin, with four handsome men following me! You could here the ladies gasping for air, and the whispering started.

"That's not MAMIE is it?" Yelled our neighbor. "Well, I'll be. I never thought she'd get one man much less 4!" I heard someone say. My head was so high and I just strolled from table to table introducing my medical school beaus, and savoring the moments. AH...R E S P E C T is so sweet. I'd finally "made it" in the eyes of the community. Whether I married any of them or not didn't matter. Mamie had her moment of glory, and I loved EVERY minute of it! This Taylor girl lost Mamie that night, and decided to keep Trix. Oh so sweet!

Of all the fun times together we had, probably the most fun was when the "whole gang" got together. On a slow weekend, brothers Dean and Gene, would join the group. Gene had by far the cutest, funniest, friends I have ever known. Being two years older, I was often included in their adventures. I see them when I go home to campaign for Gene, and they swear that all the records of those days are "locked in a vault somewhere". One of our most memorable nights was our TV debut.

Soul Train was a TV show in the 60's that came on about 11 and was one hour of bad talent acts. Groups sang, danced, did anything to get on TV. Gene and Dean got the groups together and we were "Jake the Snake" and the "Girls". Back then Go Go girls were the thing, so Sue, our friends and I tagged along as the Go Go girls. We were a little short on dancers, so we grabbed a few girls off the street to join us. We were horrible, but we were having such a good time we refused to leave. The producer literally had to carry us off so the next act could go on.

We had a ball, and we had made it to TV! All belles love EXPOSURE! Our competition had been Ruthie the Duck Woman, and the Bird whistler. Not very stiff competition now that I think about it, and we figured we had a good shot to win the prize. We had all our friends waiting up to watch us that night, including Mom and Dad. No one won the prize that night, but in reality we all won. Our ten minutes of fame. It was great!

No wonder Mom never worried about us. We were always with at least one member of the family, and the French Quarter was so safe back then. People like Ruthie and Tinkerbelle were the most "dangerous" folks that owned the Quarter. Ruthie just walked with her duck from bar to bar, talking to the locals or tourists, whoever would listen, and Tinkerbelle (the first gay guy I ever met) sold hot dogs from a Lucky Dog wagon. He certainly wasn't dangerous! Drugs may have been around back then, but we never saw them. It was just so much fun. Why did it have to end?

My two years at the LSU Medical School were some of my best years. I loved learning, I had great friends and I dated three of my med school friends. Oh yes, Mamie had fun.

I loved Mike for being so good to me. If I had had any sense at all I would have married him, but this Belle was still out for the "chase" and couldn't stand anyone being too nice. (What was I thinking?)

Busby, 14 years my senior, loved to tell me about his early years in the CIA. He really had been in the CIA and of course all I new about that was from watching

James Bond movies, so I was totally captivated! He thought I was absolutely, without a doubt THE MOST GULLABLE female on the planet. I loved it.

And Lynn, what a flirt! Anybody that calls you TRIXILLA (as if I didn't have enough nicknames!) and gave you a baby rabbit for your birthday, was too slick. He could not only make you laugh til your sides ached, but would keep you guessing as to what he was really thinking. He was lethal. We had such good times during those two years and then…. He up and married my big sister in the sorority! I was not pleased.

Partying with Jay, Sue and Duncan, Mike and Carol

7

The Learning Years

I finished my degree in physical therapy at the age of 22. I loved my profession then, and still do 30 years later. But, entering into the career world was hard. I was so sheltered and so naïve about life, the downside of being a belle.

At the appropriate time, after college, the Europe trip with Sue, and starting a career, I waited for my prince to come. I just knew it would happen because it was supposed to. I moved to a new city, Jackson, Mississippi, to establish my own identity. When you are number four of a very accomplished family, you get tired of hearing "Oh, you're Sue's sister, or Dean's sister, or one of the Taylor girls" so you break away. My time at the Baptist Hospital was enlightening, but not too much.

I loved my boss, Jim, the best physical therapist I have ever known. He was so warm, caring and out going, everyone loved him. He taught me to be a leader as well as a team player. He taught me to care and try not to get too involved. (A lesson I have never learned.) But, I was lonesome and had a hard time breaking into the "Bachelors Club" to meet people.

A year after I started working, I was engaged to "him". This tall, dark and handsome Lieutenant in the Navy cut a wide swath. He was from New Orleans, and reminded me of Rhett Butler. After five dates in a three years time frame, (can you believe this?) he proposed and I accepted. How stupid was that?

Looking back, I see that in my mind, it was my time. I had achieved all the short-term goals, got my "papers" (graduated from college), had a good job, a car and an apartment. Truthfully, I was lonely. My adventure to new territory had been successful, but there was a void. Marriage seemed like the next best step.

My "knight" needed a loving family and I really thought I could bring someone into our special family and make him happy. How little I knew. Welcome to the world Baby Belle!

We moved to Washington, DC right after the wedding and reality slowly seeped in. My first task as a military wife was to meet the other wives and learn the proper etiquette. I learned what was OK to discuss, and what was not. I was told how to speak, what to wear and who to speak too. My world began to crumble when I realized I was not in the South any more. My frequent use of the word "honey" was ridiculed, as well as my accent. I needed to change to be accepted. I didn't like it but I did it. I missed my family, my friends, and my world. I was grown up, and I didn't like it. But, I always thought it would get better. Southern women are so strong. So I lived on hope.

I knew things would get better. Four years later, we moved to Waveland on the Mississippi Gulf Coast. We bought a two story house on the beach that needed work. It was built with twelve inch concrete blocks so it would be hurricane proof and we worked like crazy on the house with a carpenter named Buddy. Three years and two baby girls later it was on the Gulf Coast Tour of Homes. I was so proud of it.

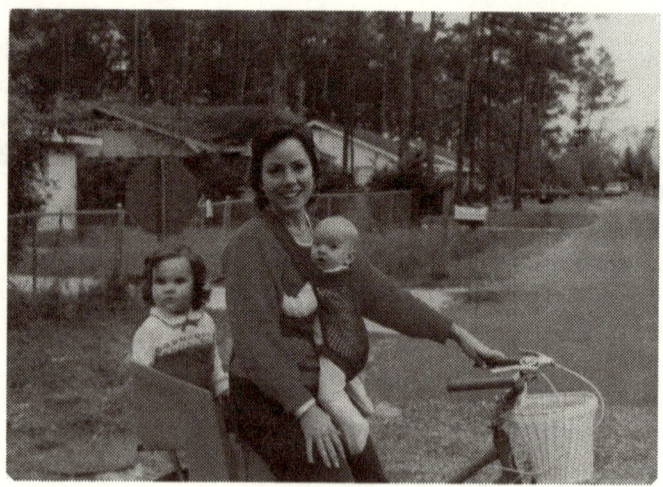

Biking with my girls in Waveland

During that time, I introduced my profession, physical therapy, to the small hospital in Bay St. Louis, a feat I am still proud of today. The doctors were great, letting me do anything I could, and to this day, I still have such respect and admiration for Dr. Sidney Chevis. Not only was he a gifted physician, but, mostly, a wonderful, caring person.

I loved working with the people of my community. Everybody knew everybody. Life was good.

My Dad was close to retiring, so Mom and Dad came over to the Bay house every weekend. I always adored him and was accused on many occasions of being "Dad's favorite". He was so optimistic. ALWAYS. His glass was always half full and he forever told me. "Things will always work out for the best". They usually did.

Dad was always so kind to under privileged people and was always giving someone a chance to make a little extra money by working in the yard or on his numerous boats.

Only my Dad would hire a young, physically, and a little mentally challenged black man to help him. Sammy was probably a thalidomide baby, for he was born with only a nub for his right arm and a contracted wrist and fingers. But, rumor had it that he was a good worker. So Sammy joined the family. He worked hard, and Mom and Dad fed him and paid him well. Then one night, Dad got a call from the police. Seems Sammy was seen around town late one night, on his bike with a TV under his nub. He was stopped and found to have not only the TV but some whiskey also. People knew Sammy worked for us so they called Dad. In the middle of the night, he went down to the jail and talked to Sammy.

Seems Sammy did steal these things from us, but Dad didn't press charges. He talked to the police and Sammy, and they sent him home. And he was back at work the next day. He worked for us for a few more years, and we never had another episode. Dad always saw the good in everyone.

Dad's passion was boating with the family, and we have such great memories of all those adventures. As with all men, "the bigger the boy the bigger the toy" theory was certainly true in our house. And in our little "water world" the toys were always boats. We used these boats to entertain friends and family, and it never failed, there was always some drama associated with our outings.

Everyone was invited on our boats, from babies to grandmas, and sometimes both. I cringe now when I think back about taking my new baby, Charlotte, on the *Calabazita*, our 32-foot sailboat. She was two weeks old, and I have numerous pictures of her and Dad and Mom on the boat. Of course, there was no life jacket in the world that would fit a newborn, but we were always confident about good weather. Right! Ask Mom how many times she called the Coast Guard! Ask Nana about our evening cruise one night.

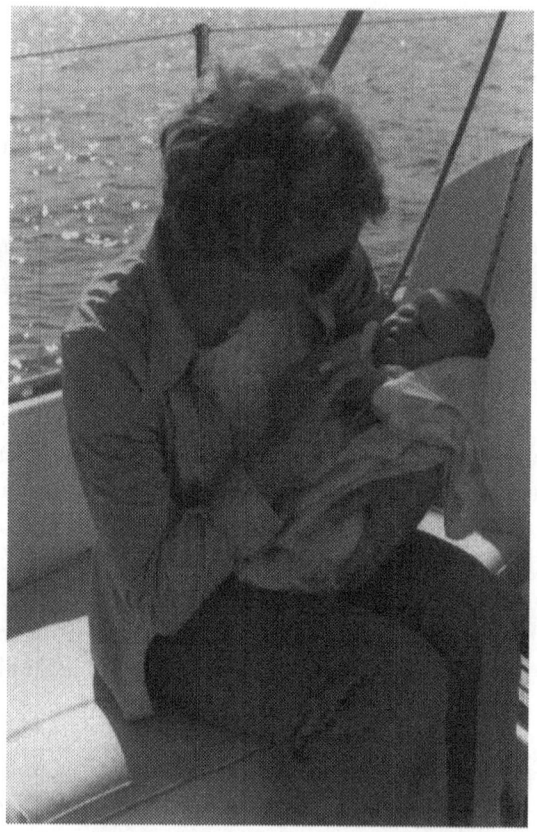

Momsy and baby Charlotte on the *Calabazita* on a good day

The weather started off beautiful, as it always did, and we took the family, Mom, Dad, Nana, my spouse and Charlotte and I, out on the Bay for a sail. We had a few cocktails on the boat, and then it hit. Only on the Bay can a squall emerge so quickly. Out of nowhere came these horrendous black clouds and gale force winds. The sails flapped frantically, and the women and children were sent below. Somehow, Nana (Mama's 88 year old mother) decided she would rather be on deck rather than maneuver the steps. Dad, wanting her out of the way, placed her on the ice chest in the middle of the boat. In this blinding rainstorm, winds howling, sails out of control, Nana glided on her own little platform from starboard to port, back and forth, soaking wet and grinning the entire time. Fortunately, she had been served a couple of cocktails prior to the storm, so she was truly floating through this entire ordeal. She laughed, as the rest of us fretted. I learned lots of life lessons from Nana, but this was the most valuable.

Lesson 7: Sometimes you just have to float through the storms.

Those were good years with the family. Even as we entered adulthood, we could be together and even help each other out.

Sue had married and moved away, so my brother, Gene and his wife, Margaret and I became very close. They lived close to Mom and Dad, and not far from me in Waveland. We were both renovating houses, living on a shoestring, and raising babies together. We rode out hurricanes together, at Margaret's parents house on Carroll Ave. always keeping our priorities, baby formula, diapers, water, flash lights, food and vodka. (For medicinal purposes only, of course).

We lived through four hurricanes in two years, boarding up the houses, moving to higher ground, and sinking the sailboat. Belles love drama and we certainly had our fair share. (Little did we know until 26 years and numerous hurricanes later, how truly devastating a hurricane can be. That safe house for us had five feet of water and mud and was uninhabitable after Katrina.)

A new dimension was added to the family one Friday evening as we gathered at Mom's house. (She fed all the families at least once a weekend. Thank God a decent meal!) My brother Gene announced that he was going to run for a seat on the City Council in Bay St. Louis. We were all dumbfounded! He was so shy, he could not even hold his head up to tell us this news flash, much less speak to a crowd of people. As a box salesman (although a Tulane grad in political science), Gene was tremendously successful on a one to one basis, but with a group? Not to mention, like us, he was just starting out and had little funds. We froze. After a few minutes to recover, we inquired who the competition might be, and when he told us, we all went silent. (A rarity in our family!)

His opponent was a very successful businessman who ran the only construction company in the town and had MONEY. How in the world could he challenge him? Not to mention, Gene was the absolute SHYEST of the entire family. How in the world was he ever going to make a speech, much less a debate?

But, we all listened to his strategy. He was going door to door, and would meet every person in his district and talk to them personally about what he could do to help the city. We were still stunned. How could he do this with a full time job thirty miles away? And no money! We didn't know anything about politics, but all we knew was it took lots of money to win elections. Or so we thought.

We rallied around him and pledged our support. If that was what he decided to do, we would support him, do whatever it took, and help him win the election. Our family always stuck together, strength in numbers, and numbers we had.

The David versus Goliath campaign began for what was to be the first of many campaigns. We rallied together on little funds, and lots of word of mouth. Then the big day finally arrived.

Mom and Margaret cooked for days for the party. We invited all the extended family and close friends that were so helpful. Those of us who were not cooking, were out passing out fliers. I had my two little girls, Charlotte, two years old, walking next to me with a "Gene Taylor for Councilman" hat on, and Liz, six months, in the stroller, with another sign on the back of it.

One of my patients, in a wheelchair from a stroke, was the head of a huge family in town. Naturally, I invited him to the party. Of course, I did this without thinking of how in the world I was going to get him to and from the party in my station wagon with two baby girls! Well, I managed and we arrived at the party just in time to see my Dad coming up the driveway with the results. I was so nervous, I couldn't breathe.

We all looked around and couldn't find Gene. He had gone out for a walk. I'll never forget that moment, when I saw my little brother walking up his driveway. Someone came screaming out of the house, yelling, "You won! You won!" The place went crazy and Gene was shell-shocked. I was not sure if he was going to "lose it" or run away, and then he took a deep breath and proceeded forward. I was so proud of him! He actually did it pretty much single handedly with some strong support from his wife, Margaret.

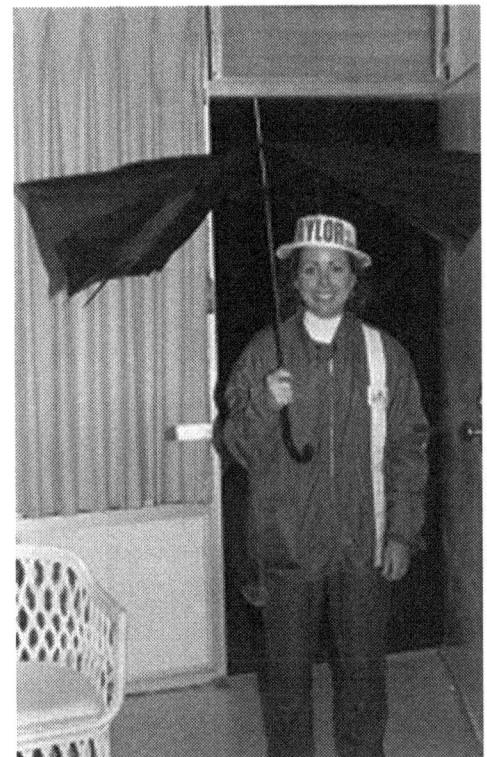

Campaigning for Gene

We were all so very proud. Another lesson learned. If you believe in yourself and persevere you can achieve your goal. This was the beginning of a long political journey for Gene. A United States Congressman for seventeen years now, he has never compromised his beliefs and has been influential in making our city, state and nation a better place. He has been tirelessly working to help the people in his area following Katrina. We are so very proud of him. A life lesson learned, and passed on to my children. All of them have been inspired by Gene's career and have achieved goals that at the time seemed impossible to reach, by persevering.

Lesson 8: Perseverance Pays Off

8

The Galvanizing Years and Men Who Need To Meet the Mafia!

Three years and two precious little girls later, (I wanted two, just like Sue and me) things should have been rosier. But they weren't. Having both my spouse's family and my family so close together turned out to be a nightmare. Of course, I wanted to be with the fun family, and he felt resentful. We worked on the house, we worked at work and we spent time with the families. We grew apart. What had I done wrong? We were supposed to live happily ever after. Reality check.

I truly believe that the number 1 reason marriages fail is that the partners grow apart, and their goals change, and they don't make the effort to stay grounded on the basic issues.

Anyway, without going into the horrible details, we grew apart and we were both going in different directions. As traumatic as it was at the time, I see now that it was the best thing for all of us. No one wins in a divorce, but after many years when the emotions are settled, lives can be renewed. I can be thankful now that I survived it, for it truly was a life challenge that ended my belle days and empowered me to make my own destiny in the real world. It gave me a new life.

Lesson 9: Divorce—Only the strong survive and reality usually hits hard.

Imagine being at home, making a peanut butter sandwich for your two year old, when your spouse of twelve years walks in and declares, "We need a divorce". "Ok" I said. Then he said, "Don't worry. I'll get the lawyer so we don't spend too much money on attorney fees." Right, and I was born yesterday.

The epiphany of my life started that day. That was mid-September 1986. This wilted magnolia, first had to deal with this situation, then perk up and become galvanized! A long row to hoe! This was, without a doubt, the hardest time in my life. Throughout all the crises in my life, (and there have been many) surviving the divorce gave me the strength to know that no matter what I had to deal with, I could make it. It took me a long time to get there, but I finally did. But first, a meltdown!

The "X" after telling the kids of our divorce, continued to live with us, in the downstairs bedroom to save money. Yes, he wanted out, but he would not leave. The slow torture began. Thus we had to endure all three holidays together, Halloween, Thanksgiving, and Christmas. A fate worse than death.

I managed to hold it together for Halloween, but by Thanksgiving I was a wreck. I cried and drank till I was bone skinny and looked 100 years old. The poor kids were so confused for they were only two, six, and seven. And we had to make it through the holidays. I needed to get it together for them, but I was so broken I needed to heal myself first.

Sue, the only family member who lived close by, was always coming to my rescue. She was so livid with the situation she couldn't see straight. I think at one point she was more upset than I was.

One day, during one of my "crazy times" Sue called with a brainstorm. She nonchalantly suggested that "the X" should be feeling a little bit of pain and that he should meet up with a Mafia guy. I couldn't believe it. The closest person in this living world to sainthood suggesting getting a "friend" to knock out both the "X's" knees! I wasn't sure if I was going to laugh or cry. "Are you out of your mind?" I asked. "You can't be serious"…But, she was. She assured me that all good folks from Louisiana have some kind of "contact" and that we could easily find ours.

God love her. Always faithful, always trying to make things better. Finally, after much discussion of the idea I convinced her that somehow I was going to pull through this without inflicting bodily harm, (much to her regret!) Divorce truly brings out the worst in people.

Although, looking back, I realize what a great idea that was, a little pain, a little bodily disfigurement, nothing too serious, and decided that was not such a bad idea after all…Some men really should meet up with the Mafia.

Lesson 10: Some men do need to meet the Mafia!

9

I Will Survive

"I Will Survive" became the theme song for the holidays that year, (and my life) and somehow I did.

Sue had the "family" over for Thanksgiving that year knowing full well what was going on and my mental status. I guess the reality of raising the kids by myself, having to work full time now, and all the responsibilities of running the house was overwhelming for me.

I wasn't sure I could do it. I didn't know the first thing about balancing the checkbook, or any automobile details. All those papers and car stickers and other mechanical things were supposed to be taken care of by the "man". This wasn't supposed to happen to me! I was supposed to live "Happily ever after". How could I work, take care of the kids and do all that stuff? I was lost in the whirlpool of life.

Anyway, our family did go to Denton with her family and her in laws. I cried the entire time. Dinner began with Sue's brother-in-law intoning a long, Thanksgiving blessing. That was it.

Somehow, through the sniffling, I finally open my eyes and look up, right into the place card holder with my name on it. I realized that those antique, floral holders had been Nana's and that Mom must have given them to her favorite, Sue. I couldn't believe it! How did Sue get those place card holders? Why didn't I get some? I was livid! As soon as the food was blessed, I proceed to give my only ally in the entire world unbelievable grief cause she got all the place card holders! That was the last straw. When I finally calmed down and Sue agreed to share with me, I realized that my old life was definitely over, and it was time for me to take charge.

Sue saw it too. She knew my out-burst was a good sign and that there was still some fire left in me and she knew, right then and there, that I was going to make it. The galvanizing had begun.

I laugh as I write this, remembering how terribly screwed up I was back then.

Divorce is just the worst for everybody, especially the children. We all know that now, and how I wish I could have done a better job at handling my transition life as well as theirs. But slowly I began to heal and then to realize my life could be a "do over".

When I look back and remember some of the things that helped me cope I find so many deeper meanings. It would be a shrink's dream to analyze some of this, so I decided to do it myself. This is what I found:

Some of the best times I had with the kids were to come home from work and watch movies. One of our favorites was *The Blues Brothers*. We would all snuggle on the couch after dinner, and when Aretha Franklin started singing "Freedom" we would all jump up and down and start dancing together back and forth in front of the TV. Well, obviously that was my theme song for the year, and I danced to it as often as I could. It still brings back good memories every time I hear it. Of course the kids had no idea of the power that song had over me. They were just glad to be up dancing with me! So, we danced a lot.

My biggest adjustment came when the kids would be with their Dad, every Tuesday, Wednesday and every other weekend. I was 35 years old and had not been alone since I was 22. I didn't know how to be alone. But, I was determined to learn.

I am so hyper that I never just "do nothing". I never just sit. I am always moving around and this was so hard for me to adjust to not having to take care of anybody. I talked to my Mom about it one day, and she said "I wonder if those pills the doctor gave me when I was pregnant with you had anything to do with you being so hyper?" I said "What, the doctor gave you SPEED when you were pregnant with me?" "Well, I just didn't have enough energy to stay up and make clothes like I used to". Was her response. Great. My Mom smoked, drank and was a Speed junkie when she's pregnant with me and I wonder why I can't sit still!

So my coping mechanism was to exercise a lot, work to remodel the house, and I finally decided to go to the movies alone. I was scared, but I did it.

Our subconscious really does kick in at the most unusual times. Like my first movie. I don't remember WHY I picked this movie, (probably cause it had three Southern women in it) but I went to see the movie *Crimes of the Heart*.

Now if you don't know this movie, it is about a petite Southern belle named Babe, who was married to a State Senator in Mississippi. The story revolves around her relationships with her husband and her two sisters.

Well for two and half hours I laughed and cried non-stop. It was great. I saw the movie three times by myself, and it was the best of all the therapies that I had. I saw myself in poor Babe, and I could laugh and cry at her messed up life, just as I was laughing and crying about my own.

I could relate so well to her. Seems Babe had enough of her mentally abusive husband and one day just up and shot him. (She didn't kill him though.) Yep, in cold blood, she just shot him! When her sister asked her why she did it, she replied, "I didn't like his looks!" This shy, timid, little woman just pulls out this huge pistol and shoots her spouse cause she didn't like his looks! I loved it! I laughed so hard I was hysterical! Then I cried. I boo hooed so loud that the people in the theater were yelling at me. I loved it so much that with every viewing I fantasized that I had up and shot my own husband too! (Divorce really puts you over the edge.) I knew I couldn't, and I wouldn't, but I loved living it through Babe. Over and over. It was great. My own little revenge. Ah...so sweet.

Then, of course, as Babe realizes the "klinker" is an option, and things start heating up, she decides life is just too much and she wants to end it all. (How many times did I feel like that too)? This was really where I could imagine myself. Unfortunately, her every crazy attempt is a failure, and the more frustrated she gets, the funnier it is.

Her first choice was hanging and this resulted in the collapse of the chandelier and the ceiling. Now walking around her house in her frilly, white sun dress, with a noose stuck around her neck, dragging the chandelier, she searches for another means of escape. (This would happen to me, no doubt in my mind.) Gas! Yes! She and the chandelier proceed to the oven for a quick gas fix. Again to no avail. As she is waiting for the oven to heat up, munching on a little leftover popcorn, she is saved by her oldest sister who is screaming, "Babe, Babe, What are you doing?" When asked why she was doing this, she gave a deep sigh and responded, "I guess I am just having a BAD Day!"

Bad Days! Oh could I relate to that! That was the story of MY life! It was ME having those bad days and fantasizing about ending it all. And just like Babe who couldn't do it because her sisters needed her, I couldn't do it cause my children needed me. Reality check. She lived through it with the help of her sisters, and I lived through mine with the help of my sister.

Of course at the time I was too messed up to figure out why I liked the movie so much but I did feel better when I came home from the movie, so I kept going. (I think it was probably the only place I could cry without being seen!)

I managed to survive those "bad days" through the love and support of my parents, old high school friend Carolina, and of course my living guardian angel, Sue.

Lesson 11: Stop Having Bad Days!

10

Courting with Children

Throughout this traumatic time in my life, I somehow managed to find humor in whatever I could. I remember talking to my patients about my life as I was treating them. I managed to use all my experiences as a diversion for all the pain and torture I was inflicting on them. They loved it. Many times they would be laughing and say, "You really should write a book." Well at the time, that was the last thing on my mind. Survival was No.1. Finalizing the divorce was No. 2

In order to finalize the divorce, the paperwork involves many hours with your lawyer. Being the naive Southern Belle that I was, I had my Daddy came in from Mississippi to help me line up a good lawyer. I am so embarrassed today as I think about that day, walking into the law office of some big shot Family Lawyer with your DADDY when you are 35 years old!

Well, this good Texas lawyer realized that there was little at stake here (relatively not much money to be had from fees) so he proceeded to direct me to his tall, blonde, good looking young partner, Larry. He strolled over, and I took one look at those blue eyes, and my heart went a racing! He looked EXACTLY like Mike, one of my old boyfriends from the medical school. I turned three shades of red and so did Larry. Things were looking good so far!

Even Dad noticed the resemblance, and with Larry a few years younger than myself, I think Dad was worried, but he listened to all the jargon and soon the deal was done. "Luscious Larry" was officially my Legal Counsel! I had a renewed will to live!

Fifteen months and three court dates later, and it still wasn't over. I had many official meetings with "Luscious", this one the most memorable. One day he called and said, "Carol, there is a problem. Can you come down here so we can talk about it?" This was no easy feat. First, it required rounding up a babysitter, and more importantly, I envisioned serious dollar signs for a one on one meeting. But, it sounded important, so I agreed.

I primped a little before I left the house; didn't want to look too bad for our meeting. As I entered his office, I looked up and saw that he was so red in the face, that I began blushing...Oh, man. "Ok, so what's going on?" I asked. Seems that when the "X" had called me the previous Friday night and I was busy, and didn't talk very long to him, he was furious. He surmised that I may have had a date and called his lawyer at home that evening to rant and rave about this divorce taking so long. Larry started laughing at this point. I was not sure if I wanted to laugh or cry. Then it hit me. As much as I liked Larry, I realized that this bickering is just a joke for these guys. They are all buddies and it is just one big happy fraternity, in this legal system of ours.

"Are you kidding?" I asked. "You brought me down here at $250 an hour to tell me that 'HE' wants to end it, cause 'He' has had enough?" I thought to myself. "Let's not forget who wanted out of here and why, not to mention it's been 15 months for me too, remember? I don't care what he does at this point."

After a few minutes I said, "Don't worry, he won't do anything stupid. He may hate me but he loves his kids. In the future, let's just chat on the phone OK?"

Larry was a good guy in a horrible profession. I cannot imagine how anyone finds fulfillment in family law unless they believe they are really helping children find a better life.

On the day (a year and a half later) we finally ended this mess, Larry told me he was going to introduce me properly to the social scene in Dallas. We had the place all picked out for me to see and be seen, and I was so excited, but as fate would have it, he was delayed with a trial and it never came to pass. That was probably for the best.

I grew stronger during that time. And to show Larry and myself what I learned from the experience, I wrote for him *Larry's Laws for the Loveless*. This I framed and asked him to display in his office so that all the other poor people who followed me, would know the REAL RULES for getting divorced. I think these RULES should be required reading for all persons undergoing this horrible time in their life. (I have attached a copy in the back of the book, just in case. You know I always like to be prepared!)

My real entrance into society began with my Coming Out Party. One day at lunch with a friend, I dropped my business card into a glass bowl for a chance to win a free happy hour for up to 100 people. You can just see the expression on my face when the phone call came that I had indeed been the lucky winner!! I seized this opportunity!

After contemplating how to maximize this windfall, Sue's nephew Whit suggested that I make this my "Coming out Party". Now remember, in those days we were still talking about Debutante coming out parties. Since I had never been, nor ever would be a debutante, we figured this was perfect. My introduction to the social scene in Dallas at the tender age of 35! So talented Whit drew up a flier with a sketch of Auntie Mame decked out in her gloves and boa, with the theme "Carol's Coming Out Party!"

I scheduled this for my weekend alone, and invited literally EVERYONE I had ever known who had been nice to me! EVERYONE! Needless to say it was a blast.

I flew white helium balloons from the front of my house as a sign to the neighbors that it was finally over. My dear ex-brother in law, Wendell, flew in to help celebrate. Tom from Michigan, Sue and Wade, my friends from work, Ranger Rick and 75 of my new best friends came to dance the night away. The "free part" ended after 1 hour, but we were all having so much fun we stayed for about four hours. Then, we proceeded on to Mexican food for the finale. I had about four hours sleep that night and I was still so excited when Wendell suggested a 5-mile run the next morning. Somehow, my adrenalin rush continued and I made it. The weekend was great fun and I was charged and ready to tackle single life again.

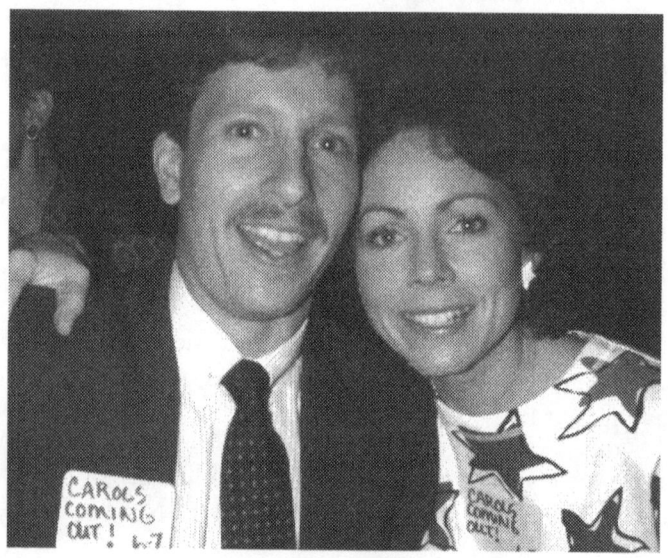

My "Coming Out Party"
Here with "Ranger Rick"

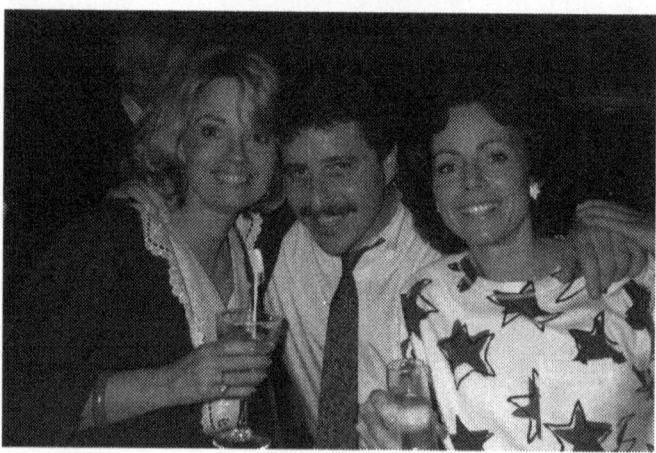

Sue, Tom Foley And Me
having fun at the party!!

I survived divorce, and my dream of living the Southern Belle life was over.

Reality check, dating in the late 1980's had certainly changed since the last time I dated back in the early 70's. Naturally, I found this out the hard way.

I was very careful when I started dating again not to include the children in any of these adventures. First of all they were dealing with enough trauma adjusting to their new "houses", and I really didn't want to get married again anyway. I had pretty much lost all faith in men, and just when I was able to take care of the kids and myself the last thing I wanted was to rock the boat with another man around. It was a great feeling to be totally independent and to know I would survive. I'd made it.

Then one day at work, one of my patients decides to rock my boat. He was a cute 29-year-old computer guy with a bad knee, and he actually started flirting with me. I treated him for a couple of weeks and as usual he knew all about my life. He got better, and when his discharge day rolled around, we happened to be walking out at the same time. He walked me to the car and asked me very casually, if I would like to go out sometime. I froze. "Like on a date?" I said. "Sure how about dinner." My facial expressions have always given me away, and I must have looked so totally shell shocked, that he started laughing. I laughed too and gave him my phone number. I got in the car and thought, "Oh My God, what have I done!"

Immediately I shifted into panic mode. Did he know how old I was? I knew he was 29 but did he know I was 35? He knew about the kids, cause I talk about them to all the patients. He would not meet the kids; better schedule this for a weeknight. What do you do on dates these days and what do you wear? I was a wreck. Then strangely enough I got excited. Somebody actually asked me out for a date! A cute guy too! Oh, but he was just a baby at 29!

After much pondering of the situation, I decided I needed a new outfit for this dinner date. I went shopping. I love to shop and had been seriously deprived for a long time so I decided it was now MY money and I could buy whatever I wanted. Boy, did that feel good! So, I bought a beautiful peach and white sweater and skirt that cost more than anything I had ever bought in my twelve years of marriage. What the hell, I was starting my new life and I needed a new look.

Date night rolled around, and I was a bundle of nerves. Got the new duds on, kids with Dad, house picked up, and I am sweating like a yard worker. Doorbell rang and I thought about vomiting, but didn't have time. I opened up the door and there he was, dressed in ironed blue jeans and a collared shirt. I felt sick. I was so totally over dressed it was embarrassing. He politely said something like, "It's just dinner," and I offered to change. Time did not permit that so I went along. Strike one.

As I walked to the passenger side of the front seat, I waited for him to come and open the door. All Southern gentleman open doors and this guy was from Arkansas, surely he knew the rules. I waited. And waited. He got in the car, then got out and said, "Are you coming?" "Oh, OK," was all I could say as I opened the door and let myself in. Strike two.

What is this deal? Men don't open the door for women in the 80's? That would take some getting used to. The date went fine. I was so worried about what these single guys were thinking going out with a DIVORCED woman. I was on high alert for any display of affection and fortunately he sensed that, so all was well.

We went out a few more times and I secretly nicknamed him "Ranger Rick" since he took me to my first Texas Rangers baseball game. He was great. He taught me how to laugh again. I found out he was seriously dating someone else, and the tension gradually eased. We talked about divorce families (his parents were divorced), the effect on kids, etc. but mostly we just laughed. I loved him for renewing my faith in men. I had been married for twelve years, had three small children, and could not remember the last time I had so much fun. I love sports, and Ranger Rick took me to sports events and on SAFE dates with lots of people around and light conversation. He was just what the doctor ordered. I was so lucky to have met him. We talked about his girl friend and he decided to get married after all. We were good for each other. I was slowly healing.

My few blind dates were disastrous. Seems all men back then were either younger than I was, or lots older with grown children. After a few dates and those "old farts" I decided a free meal was not worth it. Not to mention the thought of kissing those old birds was just too disgusting. I'd rather stay at home and read. Strike three and my dating days were over.

Then one Thursday night I received the call that would change my life forever. My friend Valerie from the clinic, called and asked if I would go to a party the next day after work to meet some of her husband's friends. This development group had just finished a shopping center and had scheduled an open house. Bottom line, they needed single women.

I gracefully declined since it was a weekend with the children. She was relentless. She called again. Her husband called and pleaded with me to come. I finally agreed to go for a little while if he promised to introduce my friend Lori and me to three eligible bachelors. Done. I arranged for the babysitter to stay an extra hour and was off to work.

No sooner had I walked into the clinic, when Lori grabbed me all excited and said she had talked to bachelors number 1, 2, and 3. She was so excited about the party. Seems these guys were playing some kind of dating game on the phone, and were asking her all kinds of stupid questions.

Ten minutes later, I get a call and this male voice announces that he is number 4, and asks what color shoes was I wearing? I laughed and it went on all day. Between patients we were getting calls from the bachelors, all six of them. By 5 o'clock we could hardly wait to meet these guys.

Within minutes of arriving at the party we had met all of the guys. This little get together was just that "little", and we were the only girls! I had no problem with that of course, and that one-hour party changed the course of my life forever. I met two very important men, one, my future husband, and two, the man who put us together.

Lori migrated to the Yankee guys since she was from Wisconsin, and I stayed with the Cajuns from Louisiana. New Orleans natives size each other up pretty quickly with one line, "Where did you go to high school?" That one answer tells you all there is to know about a New Orleanian: where they live, their financial status, and their place in society. Sometimes, though, beware, it can be deceiving!

The engineer from New Orleans, John, is a fantastic guy. Within minutes we were exchanging crawfish recipes and he was telling me what a fantastic cook his wife was, etc. He then asked me "the question" and I replied "Ursuline Academy." His eyes got the size of saucers, as he began to tease me about being from "uptown". At some point his friend came up and joined the conversation. He was introduced as No.4. My hourglass ran out and it was time to leave. John wanted to get together again and have me meet his wife sometime.

Three days later, I got a phone call from the mysterious No.4. He asked me to go to a basketball game, but I already had a blind date scheduled. I hung up the phone and thought, "Who was that guy?" I couldn't remember which one he was or what he looked like. So I called my friend. She wasn't sure either, but she thought he might be the guy from Michigan named Bob.

He called again the next week, again only introducing himself as No.4. This time I was really intrigued. Who was this guy and where was he from? I accepted the date, again on a night when the kids were gone. As the day rolled around, I needed some answers. What was his name? How old was he? (I was still hung up on age.) Did he know that I was divorced with three kids? I was a wreck. I called Valerie and asked her husband Jack to please tell me about this guy. He confirmed the name, Bob from Michigan, and age unknown, single, doubtful as to my kid status. Oh great! You walk into my house and the FIRST thing one sees are the photos of my precious children! What was I going to do? Wing it.

He comes to the door, looking so cute, and before he could say a word I proceed to blurt out in this loud frantic voice, "Do you know?" he replied, "Do I know what?" I repeat, "Do you know?" Again, "Do I know what?" "Do you know that I am divorced with three kids?" I exhaled out. There was a slight pause and he responded, "I heard that you had been around the block a few times!" That was it. He was OK. I laughed so hard, opened the door and let him in. The beginning of a new life with laughter.

Lesson 12: A second chance—Go for it!

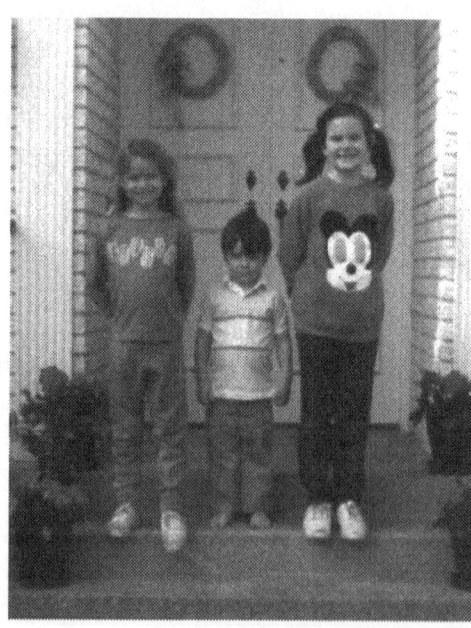

My precious children: Elizabeth age 7, Ed age 3, and Charlotte age 8

11

Oh No, Not A Yankee!

A few weeks later, after a several dates, I still hadn't figured out this Bob guy. Yes, he was a Yankee, but I was trying to accept all different kinds of people. He had worked in Houston when everyone left Michigan in the 80's, and recently was transferred to Dallas.

We went on "safe dates" to sporting events, and after meeting with his boss I began to wonder about his age. His boss was so young, I thought, oh no, not another baby! But, age never came up so we just cruised along very slowly.

We did meet again with John, the friend from New Orleans. Seems like John was so impressed with the fact that I went to an "uptown" private school that he convinced Bob that I must have money and he needed to date me. Boy was he off base! But John deduced that I was from the ritzy part of New Orleans and now lived in a house in the "bubble" part of Dallas, so I must have money. I howled when I heard this. Rich? Are you kidding? Men are so easily impressed. I was definitely rich, rich in children, but that was the extent of it. I teased him a lot about that. I must say, Bob was disappointed when he heard the news, but fortunately, he still asked me out.

I was afraid to get involved, so we dated casually for a few months when the kids were with their Dad. Poor Bob, I drilled him constantly about his life, family and their relationship. I was trying so hard to be smarter and really learn as much about him. I was determined not to make the same mistake twice.

I was still analyzing Bob, when a situation arose that I couldn't handle by myself.

One of my patients died, and the family wanted me to attend the funeral. This is a therapist's worst nightmare. We work with the living and, no matter what the diagnosis, we always keep a positive attitude and strive to be upbeat with our treatment approach. I knew this patient had a terminal brain tumor, and we had established a close bond, but I was not prepared for his early demise. I never went to funerals. I always like to remember the patients having fun working with me, and so I declined when his wife called.

It was a request I really wasn't ready to handle just yet. My mental status was less than stable, and I did not trust a chance for a serious emotional release like this. Then she told me how much I meant to her husband in those last months and that she wanted to say that at the funeral and she wanted me there to hear it. I was stunned. No, no, not a funeral! I agonized about going for days until my friend Valerie suggested that I ask Bob to go with me for moral support.

"You can't be serious, ask him to go to a funeral? Who in their right mind goes with a date to a funeral?" I replied to Val. But, I was desperate. I had an obligation to the family and I couldn't let my weakness dictate my life, so I asked him. He agreed. Bob picked me up and saw that I was as pale as a ghost. I was trying hard to hide my nerves, but my hands were shaking so much, and I was so upset I couldn't keep still. Realizing I had failed to eat, he took me to get a quick bite before we went to the church.

It was without a doubt one of the longest hours of my life. We sat on the back row, and I "tuned myself out" so I wouldn't start crying. Then my patient's wife started talking about our time in therapy. The tears trickled down my cheeks, and they wouldn't stop. I blinked, I breathed deeply, I squeezed my hands, but nothing eased the sadness or controlled my emotions. I could not escape from them. Then, without warning, Bob reached over and took my hand in his. He didn't say anything, and he didn't look at me. He just held my hand. It was so warm and strong. He had never held my hand before and I was so touched by this small gesture of support. I looked up at him and it hit me…this is a very special man. I finally got it right.

Our relationship changed that day. I wasn't afraid to let someone else in my life, and so we both took a leap of faith and let down the barriers. I found out he was five years younger than me! My heart sank. I waited for the old brush off, but he said he had no idea how old I was and that it didn't matter. Was he for real?

We were so different. I am so hyper and he is so calm and methodical. I say thirty thousand words a day to his thirty. I loved the South and warm weather, while he was used to Michigan's cold. He works with things, I work with people. He balances the checkbook to the penny, and I loose the statements! He fixes things and

I hate all mechanical things. I get lost in the neighborhood, and he loves maps. We were both so strong in some respects and so weak in others. Strangely enough, we found we could compliment each other! After four months, we were serious enough that I felt comfortable introducing him to the rest of the family. We would try to have these two different halves blend into one and see if we could raise a "ready made" family together.

12

We are Family!

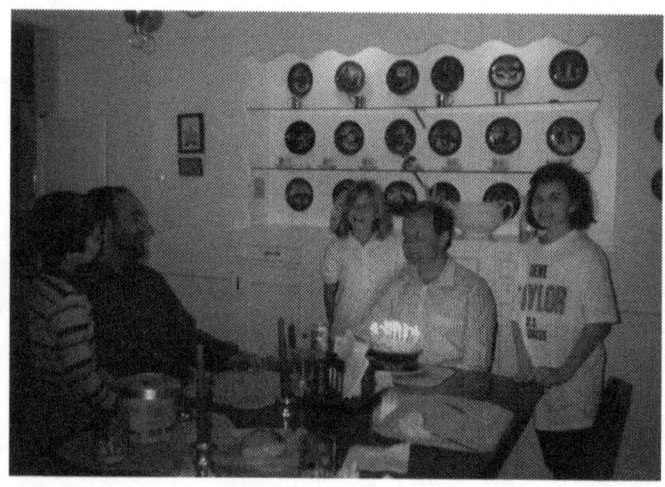

Bob's birthday party, three weeks after he proposed to me. Ed, John, Liz, Bob and Char

Can you imagine what it must be like for someone who has never been married or had kids to start dating a woman with a three year old boy and seven and eight year old girls?

I wish I had a picture of the first time Bob came to the door to pick me up when the kids were home. My babysitter had put those cute pink sponge rollers in Charlotte and Liz's hair. When the doorbell rang, all three kids ran to the door. Charlotte, the oldest, opened the door and standing at attention, like little stair steps were these three precious children dressed for bed. "Is your Mom here?" he asked. They all started giggling and running around screaming, "He's here, he's here". After a quick beer (a little liquid courage) we said our goodbye's (the traumatic part) when Ed came up to me and said, "Momma how come I can't have rollers in my hair too?" Bob gave me this shocked look and I proceeded to say that he could if he wanted them. We got to the car and Bob looked at me and asked, "Is that normal that little boys want rollers in their hair?"

Oh, he had a lot to learn! And learn he did.

Unfortunately for him, but fortunately for me, the development company Bob worked with went "belly up" a few months later. This was happening a lot in Dallas in the late 80's, and he was happy with the severance pay, so he wasn't too distressed. (He never got too distressed back then…I did enough for both of us!)

So, somehow, Bob just started helping out. He would come over in the mornings and find out who needed to be where, and what my work schedule was like and we began sharing the responsibilities. Before I knew it, he was running all the car pools, attending all the soccer games and staying home in the afternoon with Ed. He was great! The kids got a chance to know him without me around and he started making time to be with each one alone so he would know them better.

I'd call from work and he'd proudly report that he and Ed had been watching the TV show Mr. Ed, finished lunch and that Ed was down for his 1:00 nap. Wow! He then decided that it was time to redo my handiwork around the house. In my "therapy time" when the kids were first gone to their Dad's I remodeled the interior of the house. But, my way and the engineer's way were very different. I did the quick fix version and Bob only does things PERFECTLY. So, my feelings were not hurt when he offered to really paint the house and put in new carpet. And he did.

Six months went by, with the same routine. Mr. Mom comes over in the morning, stays until after dinner and went home at eleven. Ed started calling Bob "Dad" and of course the "X" went ballistic. Liz was crazy about him and craved the attention. My precious first-born Char was the most traumatized at age nine and wanted her old life back. But, she saw that I was happier when Bob was around and she liked that.

I finally met Bob's family after seven months of dating, at his sister's wedding. It wasn't until after I got to Michigan that I learned that Bob hadn't really mentioned that I was divorced with three kids. I was livid! How do you NOT mention this piece of information? You're dating an older, divorced woman with three kids and you fail to mention this?

Seems he wasn't sure how his Mom, a very devout Catholic, would react to this news. So, I make it through the ceremony, sitting with the in-laws and trying hard not to mention my kids. NO WAY! I tried not to talk much, and when I did, I inadvertently talked about them during the entire dinner. After two very awkward hours, little wine (his Mom doesn't approve of drinking) Bob came and rescued me. Out in the yard, I lost it. I was hysterically crying. My children are, and always will be, the most important part of my life, and to pretend like they are not there was just awful. Bob apologized and admitted his fears.

We left Michigan with Bob assuring me he would talk to his family and there would be no more surprises. His Mom was so wonderful, and loved it later on when I told her we called Bob, "St. Bob". The family was very understanding, and have since welcomed my family into theirs.

Then, the real test: Meet the Family Part Two.

Being the avid Southerner that I am and wanting my spouse to not only believe in the South but relish its fine qualities, I insisted on a mini road trip through our fair region to show him the finer parts of our country.

One long holiday weekend, when the kids were with their Dad, Bob and I took off to meet the folks. We were pretty sure that a merger was eminent, so he needed to understand my roots. Our first stop from Dallas was Vicksburg, Mississippi. We toured the battlefield and stayed in a beautiful Bed and Breakfast that had been an old plantation. It was gorgeous. Bob was such a good sport through all of this, and he never complained.

Next, we were on to Natchez. Again more battlefields and more mansions. As I drooled over all the fabulous homes, he followed two steps behind. Another fabulous old Southern plantation home for the night, and by the end of the day though, he did have to remind me that the South did lose the war! Why are men so practical? A few viewings of *Gone With the Wind* would straighten him out!

We finally arrived in Bay St. Louis and it was meet the family time.

Mom had been cooking for days, and the entire entourage was there to meet the "new boyfriend". It was crazy. Brothers and sisters, nieces and nephews, adopted aunts and uncles. Poor Bob, he wasn't sure who was real family and who was adopted family! We ate seafood and drank wine til the wee hours. It was chaos, and he had survived the first test.

The next day, was campaign day. Gene had lost a bid for US Congress the previous year to a local sheriff who was killed in a plane crash a few months after taking office. Now Gene was running again for the seat. So, the family pulled together again for another campaign.

Bob was assigned to go with Uncle Henry (an adopted uncle) to the back woods of the Bay and install yard signs. The girls were strategically located at different shopping centers handing out push cards. We convened at 9 am and would meet up again at 6. This was serious business.

Bob loved Uncle Henry. Uncle Henry was Dad's best friend. He and his wife, Elsa, were friends with Mom and Dad before I was born back in the fifties. They played together, and they suffered together. Uncle Henry was always just one step away from "the big deal" that would make him rich. He tried all types of options from playing the ponies, developing real estate, investing in wonder pills, or selling whatever the latest gadget was at the time.

When he hit it big, he was the most generous man in the world. I remember one day when I was about five. He drove up to our Bay house on Second Street, in a beautiful black thunderbird convertible. All of us kids raced to see him and drool over his car. As he stepped out of his car, he had presents for us. (He had no kids at that time). We were going through some tough times and presents were rare. He had bought shoes for all of us! We were so excited. Yes, when things went well for Uncle Henry he was so generous. Unfortunately he failed to save for a rainy day, and those days came real soon.

Dad and Henry had the kind of friendship that warms your soul. Uncle Henry was always my date in high school for the Ursuline father/daughter dance. Dad had two daughters for that dance, so Uncle Henry was always willing to pitch in for me. We would dance and carry on. He was great.

Dad and Henry grew old together. When his wife had had enough of the unstable living, he moved to the Bay to be close to us. He was a helluva fisherman and a pretty good boatman, so he was in on all of our boat trips. The last boat trip Dad, Henry, Steve, and I took together was so typical.

We take off and it is sunny on our side of the Bay, and cloudy on the Pass side. When Henry was a little reluctant about taking my brother's old shrimp boat across the Bay for gas, Dad blasted at him, "Oh Baltar, it's not going to rain, that squall will go around us." Famous LAST words! We head out of the harbor, cruising along at bird speed (slowly), and make it to the gas dock. The clouds had become dark gray and black, but Dad, our Captain, was not worried.

As we headed back home, in a flash, the rain comes down in buckets. "Turn on the wipers, Dad," I yell over the roar of the motor. "What?" "The wipers. I can't see out the windows, can you?" Nope. He couldn't see either! "They don't work. Carol, you and Henry get up there and tell me when you see another boat or the lines of the crab traps."

Steve leans over to me and asks, "Mom are we going to die?" I lied in reply, "No honey. We'll be fine: it's just a little storm." To this day I HATE thunderstorms and will not leave the house in one. Dad was yelling at Henry, and next thing I saw was Henry taking something out of his mouth and putting it in his pocket. We forged ahead, slowly, through the blinding rain. Dad, Henry and I are soaking wet, since we have to navigate from the porthole.

Mom, of course saw the storm coming from our house and tried calling us. Dad forgot the phone. The radio on the boat was broken too, (surprise, surprise) so we were "incommunicado." She finally took off driving down the coast until she spotted us and literally followed us back to the harbor. When we got off the boat, Dad looked at Henry and noticed his teeth were missing! "Good Heavens, Henry, where are your teeth?" At that point I recalled seeing Henry put something in his pocket, and began laughing. Seems Henry puts his teeth in a safe place when he got nervous! "Put your teeth in your mouth, you look like an old fool!!" Dad scowled. Dad always gave Henry grief, and vice versa. We all laughed. Every time I see those "Grumpy old Men" movies I think of Dad and Henry. That was how Dad and Henry were. They loved each other so much and had such a special bond.

Over the years Henry's illnesses mounted and when the shakes got real bad we insisted he see another VA doctor. We later learned that it wasn't the lack of vodka and tea that gave him the shakes, it was Parkinson's disease! His trusty timer would signal "pill time" and Henry would dash for his stash! What a character!

Henry was also one great historian. His family had roots in Mississippi for generations and he shared these stories with Bob on the sign-pounding excursion. His big claim to fame was his cousin from Biloxi, Fred Haise, who flew on the Apollo 13 space mission.

After a weekend of family talk, campaigning, and interrogation, Bob was approved and thus christened by my Mom as "St. Bob." They were so excited for me for they could see how truly happy I was, and what a great man Bob was to marry a woman with three kids. Not to mention he was so good to me! I was so lucky. Our family embraced him that weekend, and they would later find out how truly special he was.

13

St. Bob

Weeks turned into months, and daily we all learned more about each other. Bob was so good and so funny. He had so many new things to learn about kids. He had assumed they just "knew things". Like, cutting your food. At any meal if we had anything that required cutting, I would just go around the table and proceed to cut all the children's food. He would look at me and say, "Why are you cutting their food?" All Moms know that kids are slow to cut and it takes you about two seconds to do it, and them about five minutes. So although the girls were quite capable of cutting, I did it anyway because I was faster.

This would not fly with Bob. "This is the reason you are so exhausted at night", he would say. "Let them help you." The kids froze. Their free ride was over. What? Not only did he dismiss my cutting activities, but he also began delegating chores for everyone.

Now, I would never have done that. It just took too much energy to fight with them about helping, and it was easier for me to just do it myself. But, Bob was raised with the chores and routine approach and he gradually implemented some of it into our life.

Every Saturday, the kids helped clean the house. They really didn't complain much for he always bribed them with some special outing. Whatever works!

After about a year of dating, I start putting the pressure on for a serious commitment. Bob was so scared. One night at dinner with our friends, John started giving Bob grief about getting married, and the poor guy was so freaked out he stayed in the car! We are all in the restaurant ordering cocktails wondering what had happened to Bob. He had gone to park the car and then the severity of the moment set in and he froze. After about ten minutes John went to check on him. He came back into the restaurant shaking his head and laughing. "He said he was just thinking, and would be in shortly." An hour later, (we ate without him,) he dragged himself in complaining of an upset stomach. "You don't mean NER-VOUS stomach, do you BOB?" asks John. "Maybe," he confessed. So, we let up. He would make a move on his own schedule, not ours.

A few months later, we planned a weekend to Taos. It was October and I had never been there. Bob assured me it would be beautiful with the fall colors. So we flew to Albuquerque, and drove through the mountains to Taos. It was truly spectacular—the colors so vivid, the sky so blue, and the air so crisp. It was beautiful. As we drove through this picturesque scene, I noticed that Bob was more quiet than usual, (only ten words that day!) but, I just assumed it was the drive and that he was tired.

The next morning he announced that we were taking a hiking trip up the mountain.

"Hiking? Are you serious?" I was in fairly good cardiovascular condition. Bob had been, before he met me and started eating with us. Now it was ice cream every night for him and the kids, so you can imagine what kind of shape he was in! But he convinced me that he was in better shape than I thought, and off we went.

I had never hiked before in the mountains and the combination of the altitude, and the incline was a real eye opener for me. So we went up, and up, and I asked, "How much farther? My back is starting to hurt!" "Just a little farther. There is something up here I want you to see, and the view is great."

Twenty more minutes," Are you sure there is something up here? I'm getting pretty tired." I said. "A little farther" he says. After another thirty minutes I'd had it. Hot, sweaty, out of breath, and nothing to see but trees. "That's it, I am NOT going another step. I've had it. This is not fun, this is WORK!" I proclaimed. "OK, we'll stop here. You thought I was in bad shape!" He proceeded to give me grief. Then he took off his jacket and laid it on the dirt, and sat down. "Come sit by me." He motioned toward the jacket. I sat, closed my eyes and tried to breathe. In a flash, he was on his knees, looked up at me and asked me to MARRY HIM! "What?" I was so dumbfounded! "What did you say?" He pulled a little bag out of his pocket with a beautiful diamond set in a temporary setting, and handed it to me. I was speechless! (a rare moment for me) and I start crying (my usual response to intense happiness or sadness). I felt ashamed of complaining non-stop for the past hour, and gave him a big hug. "Of course, I will. Are you sure your ready for this?" I ask. "Here I try to provide the perfect setting to ask you, on top of the mountain, next to a lake, and you bitch and moan the entire way up! Not to mention I haven't slept in days I've been so nervous about this!" I began laughing, "I'm sorry. If I'd have known I would have cooperated a little more. No wonder you haven't said but three words all weekend!"

I was elated. We got off the mountain and drove to the nearest pay phone (the Safeway Supermarket) and I called Mom and Dad. They were thrilled. Bob decided he needed a little bit of "fortification" before he would call his folks, and so waited until that night at dinner. The beginning of my second life started that day, this time with a real prince. I was so happy.

The hardest part of instant fatherhood for Bob was the personal hygiene part. He never quite got the hang of wiping! Yep, the big obstacle of parenthood was wiping children's bottoms!

The day we got back from our trip, I took the girls to help me pick out an engagement ring setting (he wanted that to be a girl thing), got home and found him frazzled.

Seems Ed had to do "the big one" and upon completion began to sing out "Come wipe me…Come wipe me." Now he was three years old, right? Out of diapers but not proficient with cleaning the bottom. So, like all good Moms, I did it. But, I wasn't there! Bob finally tracked down the singing, and found Ed in the bathroom. When Ed saw Bob he dropped his head to the floor, and put his hands on his ankles.

Bob walked in to see Ed's little bottom staring him in the face and he GAGGED! Frantically he says to Ed, "What are you doing?" "You need to wipe me" was the response. "Oh no. I don't do that." "But Mom's gone." Bob desperately tried to think of another out. "Do I really have to?" Ed nodded. Being the good engineer that he was he analyzed the situation and determined that his problem was not the deed to be done, but the odor of the deed to be done. So, he searched through all the bathrooms until he found the right remedy: Vicks Vapo Rub! A big hunk under the nose and all other odors are history. Finally after ten minutes of stalling the deed was done. Bob always found a clever way through a tough situation!

When I got home the first question was, "How old are kids when they can wipe themselves?" Poor baby. He had a whole lotta learning to do!

After a year of dating, we decided to do it. We were trying very hard to make everyone happy. I applied for the annulment a few months after my divorce, and after eighteen months was told they had no clue where I was on the list. By December, Bob had taken a new job, and we were ready to move on as a family. The Church was not cooperating, so we decided we would get married by the Justice of the Peace and when the annulment came through, the Church would bless us.

Our big day arrived, December 17, the day before my parent's anniversary. I had bought red satin dresses with big white collars for the girls, Ed had a little red blazer and a bow tie, and I had an off white suit. Bob was so nervous, he didn't want too many people so we only had our friends, John and Maureen, and my sister Sue and her kids. We decided that we wanted the kids to have a fun day, too, so each child was allowed to invite one guest for the afternoon.

After the wedding we took all the kids, in their nice clothes, to the local establishment, Dave and Busters, for hamburgers and video games. We stayed there for 3 hours and Bob gave the kids lots of tokens. They played games and they had a ball. It was great. This was a different kind of reception for sure, but one where everyone had a good time.

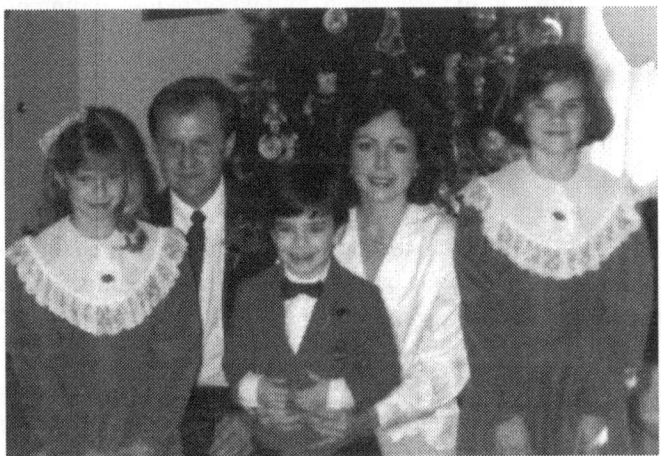

Our wedding day December 17, 1988

Our friends watched the children that night for our honeymoon, and the next day at noon Bob moved in. Our blended family and my second life finally became official. I thanked God, for I knew I was the luckiest woman in the world, and I had been blessed with the life lessons to survive even the most devastating challenges.

Life is never the same after a divorce. You can either fight it or accept it. We decided to accept it and try to make new traditions, rather than moan about not having the old ones.

Holidays are by far the hardest times in blended families. New traditions are crucial, and hard to implement. It means sacrificing what you would like to do, and do what is best for your "first" family. Our annual Christmas trips to the Bay were out of the question. Our divorce decree made sure of that. We were the only family among my siblings who rarely made it home for Christmas. We didn't make it to Michigan either, so we did the best we could at home. We learned to make it work.

The annulment finally came through and we had our families in for the blessing of the marriage and a big party. We had it at Sue's house and it was lots of fun. The families got together and, finally, the North met the South.

Two months later, at the tender age of 38, I discovered I was pregnant! We were all so excited! Bob was thrilled, Ed was thrilled, Liz was thrilled and Char was a little embarrassed. After all she was eleven, and we were just finding out how difficult those middle school years were.

The girls and I shopped for maternity clothes, and Ed just wanted a baby brother. The big decision about the amniocentesis came up and I had very mixed feelings. Bob was for it, and my gynecologist neighbor finally persuaded me. So I had the test, and we waited. Two weeks later, the results were back and it was indeed a healthy baby boy! Oh, we were all so excited. We went to TGI Fridays to celebrate and to have a name the baby party. We all liked Scott, and since Bob's middle name was Joseph we went with Scott Joseph. It was a done deal. Or so we thought.

Two weeks later, I went in for a routine checkup. I was about 26 weeks along. The nurse practitioner couldn't find the heartbeat. "Oh, it's there," I said, "We just got the test results and he is just fine." "Well let's take you down for a sonogram to be sure."

Fine, I was on top of the world. Being a department supervisor, I knew all the people in X-ray and just breezed in for the test. A temporary technician did my ultrasound and within minutes called for a physician. Two minutes later, the doctor proceeded to tell me that there was no heartbeat and that my baby had died. Just like that. "That can't be," I said. "Keep looking, keep looking. I see him. He's fine." "Babies are a miracle, Carol, and yours didn't make it." He left the room.

The sweet technician asked where my husband was and what was his number. I lay there in shock, refusing to believe this guy. "Try again, please someone look again" I heard myself saying. But I was alone. There are no words to explain that horrible feeling.

Minutes later, Bob arrived. We just cried. How can this be? What did I do wrong? The tests just said he was OK. What happened? It was awful. And it got worse.

My doctor finally arrived, and said something about delivering the baby, but there were no rooms available. I had to go home and come back tomorrow. This was a major hospital, and there were no beds? Or was it just no beds for HMO patients?

We went home and faced the children. It was terrible. How do you tell children that babies just die? Someone has to take the blame? What happened? The girls went on to their soccer games and I found out later, cried to their Dad about my losing the baby. Ed was six years old and just snuggled up to me and wouldn't stop crying. It was truly one of the worst nights of my life. And poor Bob, he was so upset yet he had to be so strong. We had difficult decisions ahead.

Our baby boy was delivered the next day. Mom, Dad and Sue were there with Bob for loving support. They never left my side. My sister Di lost her baby boy years earlier and encouraged me to see the baby. When I finally saw him, as drugged up as I was, I will always remember his eyes. He was so tiny, about the size of your hand, and he had the most beautiful crystal clear blue eyes, just like Bob's. The hospital somehow failed to take a picture of him, so we left empty handed. Fortunately, I will always have the memory of that tiny little miracle with those beautiful blue eyes. I survived death.

Ten years later, I am now volunteering at a large hospital where I feed and rock neonatal intensive care babies. I see babies as small as mine were, that are now surviving. I think about my little baby boy and wonder about him. It wasn't time for my little angel, Scott, and I am comforted to know that I have a precious little angel waiting to meet me one day, when the time is right.

Two months later, the time was right, and I was pregnant again. With this pregnancy I demanded a high-risk specialist. At 39, having been on bed rest for four months with Ed, losing Scott, and now pregnant again I didn't have time for any more mistakes.

The specialist reviewed my past history and determined that our first baby died from a slow acting infection from the amniocentesis. I was shocked, and relieved. Relieved to know that it wasn't my fault. I was placed on antibiotics and had numerous ultrasound tests during my pregnancy. I was a nervous wreck for nine months. I was still working and so paranoid that I would slip into the ER, between my patients and use their fetal monitor every day to make sure his little heart was still beating. No amniocentesis, this time, just faith in God.

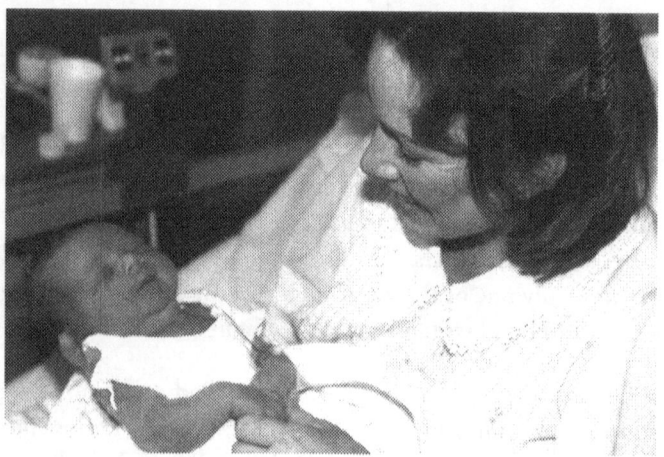

Steve's birthday, February 7, 1991

Our little miracle, Stephen Robert, was born almost eleven months to the day after we lost Scott. God wanted him here for us. Steve was the love of the family. The girls and I fought over who got to feed him, and Ed just adored him. Bob was in heaven. He had started his own business and was very busy when Steve was one, but managed to come home and play with the kids every night, then go back to work after they went to bed.

Before we knew it, we had teenagers and a two year old. The girls were busy with ballet, gymnastics and piano, and Ed with sports. We dragged Steve to all the events, and everyone spoiled him. We bought a custom van for the family with TV and VCR. It was time for the "family vacation".

I love those Chevy Chase vacation movies. They are so hysterical. Some of our trips could be used as part of the next script! With our children's ages so spread apart, it was hard to find something that everyone wanted to do. But, we tried.

Our first ski trip in the van was when Steve was a year old. We took off in the middle of the night for New Mexico, and made it by the next afternoon. Not two miles away from our resort, we took a wrong turn. By this time all the kids are screaming, "How much farther?" "We're almost there," I replied. Then it happened. Steve was in the middle seat in his car seat with the three in the way back lying down watching a movie. With every little whimper, the girls gave Steve another bottle of milk, so by the time we hit the altitude, motion sickness set in. He started projectile vomiting and all the kids froze, and then screamed. I jumped across the seat in time to spring him from the car seat before he aspirated. But not before he had hit all the food, the tapes and inside the VCR. It was horrible! The smell of sour milk all over Steve, me, and the back of the van was disgusting. The kids hid under a blanket to keep from seeing the mess. Typical!

We finally arrived at the condo only to be told that the room wasn't ready. I lost it. How could we wait another hour in this smelly van? We certainly couldn't go into a restaurant like this. So, I took charge. I walked in with my sick baby and begged for the use of a bathtub for a quick fix. One whiff of Steve and me was all it took. We were escorted to a room and were able to clean up a bit. Bob joined us shaking his head. The van was a nightmare. He escorted the family to the restaurant, we ate, and he and the kids went to clean the van. What a saint!

Bob's business was growing, so I decided to leave my part time, supervisors job at an out patient clinic, and go back to working home health where the hours are really flexible.

That lasted for a year, and I felt I needed to be a little more productive. So, another bit of fortune happened. I found the most wonderful orthopedic surgeon to work for. I worked part time, three days a week, and still had time to get home for the kids and the activities.

The proud grandparents, Bob and Margaret Lander, Penny and Gary Taylor

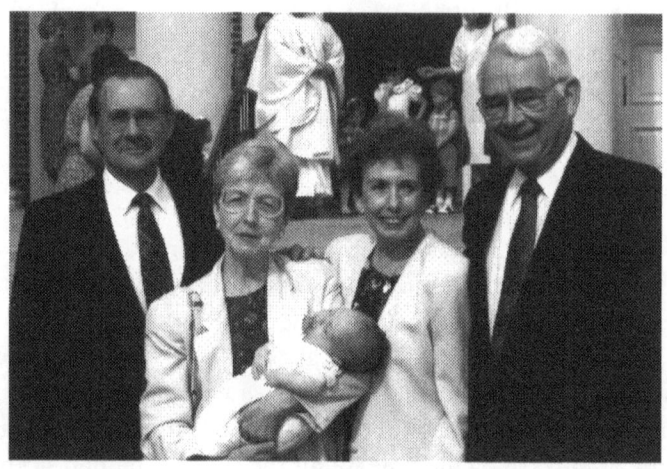

14

Another Crisis: The Big C

In November of 1995, following my annual check up, I realized that my doctor, who was also my friend, failed to say anything about a mammogram. So, I called the office when I got home and they apologized for their error. Yes, I needed a mammogram. I had the test and as I was walking out the door, they called me back. "We just want to do one more thing." Are you kidding? This could have come right from the script of the Murphy Brown show.

"I do not have time for this, bla, bla bla, and I have NO boobs, how can I have cancer?" I arrogantly answered. Anyway, they did the ultrasound and then recommended a biopsy. "Look, I have no history in the family, it's the holiday time, can't this wait till after the first of the year?" So, they agreed. I didn't think about it again for two months.

I had the test on January fourth, and I waited. I am such an optimist that it really never occurred to me that this might actually be a problem. Not until I phoned the doctor's office and no one would give me the test results.

By two in the afternoon, and three phone calls later, still no word from the surgeon. I finished with my patients and then the phone rang. It was the surgeon who proceeded to tell me OVER THE PHONE that I had ductile carcinoma insitu. What? "Say that again?" I heard myself say. She repeated and then said, "You have breast cancer and I need to see you and your husband in my office in the morning at ten. Bye." I put down the phone, and sat still. What was going on here? Did she say Cancer? Breast cancer? I walked across the hall to the orthopedic clinic and announced, "I have breast cancer. The doctor just called and told me." Silence. My orthopedic doctors stared at me, and I kept walking.

I knew this was bad, but I couldn't think about it now. I needed to go home and take care of Steve, now almost five, and see about the girls. I just couldn't think about that now. Later. Later I will think about it. It'll be fine. Everything is going to be fine. I proceeded to cope by thinking this is not happening to me but to one of my patients. If it were my patient, I'd say, "Don't worry, everything is going to be fine." So I said it to myself.

I walked in the back door, and Bob was waiting for me. We hugged and he cried. "It's going to be OK," I said. "Don't worry." But he did worry, much more than I did, then.

One of his colleagues was a real estate broker who had just been through all this. She had a mastectomy and chemotherapy, and Bob had seen her struggle with the treatment. He envisioned me, suffering like Karen did. He called and told her, and she immediately set us up with her cancer doctor for a second opinion.

Mom and Sue came in and took over. The support troops went to work. I knew a fair amount about many aspects of medicine, but knew zero about breast cancer. We talked to all friends, doctors and family and got numerous opinions. It was overwhelming. The doctor always wants to move quickly, and thus we really had no time to think. Diagnosis confirmed, surgery scheduled. Lumpectomy and radiation. I hope I made the right decision.

At 45 years of age with two teenage daughters, an adolescent son and a five year old, it was hard to truly deal with the possibility of death. As a Catholic, I felt like I had strong faith, but never really thought much about my own mortality. So denial seemed my best coping mechanism. I didn't talk about it to any of the children, for I didn't want to get them upset. I couldn't talk about it, so I read about it. I became an expert.

Dr. Phil (who is the only shrink I really like) says, "Monsters live in the dark". How true that turned out to be for me. Unbeknownst to me, monsters were hiding around my family. I finally proceeded with work and radiation, after numerous problems. It never fails; people who work in the medical field do have the worst luck when they are patients.

It just amazed me at how uncaring the medical profession can be. So often patients are basically treated like a number with little or no regard for the "whole person". And doctors say the dumbest things! My oncology team, after scientifically locating the exact area to radiate with their fancy machines, used a black (or red or green) marking pen to outline the area to be treated. A marking pen! I don't even want to get started on the accuracy of this method, not to mention the humiliation for the poor patient. Imagine that a big black square has just been placed around your entire boob with two x's. Now the technician tells you not to wear anything that will disturb the marks, (forget Victoria's Secret lingerie) and not to wash off any of the marks for six weeks. You heard right! No water on your breast for six weeks. "Now go home and forget you have cancer!" I kid you not. That was exactly what happened. I was stunned! Were these people for real?

Most were so used to seeing this, and of course they did not have cancer. I was so sensitive, but I was looking for a little more empathy. I don't know how the others handled it, but I sure didn't like the reminder. So I would change in the dark to avoid looking at the black box and hoped Bob would never see it.

March rolled around, and our family trip with Steve, Mom, Dad, Rosie (our adopted sister) Sue and her family to Mexico neared. I desperately needed a mental health check. Between working, writing, daily radiation treatments, and taking care of the family, I was exhausted. I was still in denial, so that was even more draining.

So, I asked the technician for a weekend pass, and that was granted. Upon inquiring where we were going, she immediately started listing the things I could not do while on this trip. No sun, no swimming, no snorkeling (my favorite things to do in the world) no getting the marks wet, remember? That was it. I lost it big time. I was hysterically crying. I had to escape this constant reminder of death and cancer. Five weeks of seeing people struggling to survive, my own façade that "I was fine", and running crazy in my own life, hit me hard. The technician was very sweet, and agreed that it would be OK to swim with lots of sunscreen, and that the marks could be replaced. "The doctor can re-mark you when you get back. They just don't like to. Whatever you do, don't say that I told you that." A much-needed reprieve was in sight.

We had a great few days. Bob and I truly enjoyed being with the family, and we finally had a few minutes to somehow deal with what was going on. Monday rolled around way too fast, and I was back in radiation. A different technician took one look at my faded marks and "went ballistic". After a few minutes of bustling around and many upset staff members, a doctor FINALLY agreed to re-mark me. This took all of three minutes. THREE minutes of their precious time under those sophisticated machines, and I they gave me hell cause I lost the markings! I was livid. I left that day resolved to be sure that before my eight weeks was up the director of the department would hear about how patients are treated.

The sad part is they really didn't care.

Another lesson learned.

Lesson 13: Take charge of your medical care and Find a doctor who truly cares about you.

Not long after, at a birthday party for one of Steve's friends, I met a nice man who listened very attentively to my cancer horror stories and then proceeded to tell me that his wife was a breast cancer surgeon at the Medical School! My angels had intervened again. I called her and went for a follow up. She was fabulous. I transferred all my paper work to her and for the first time, I felt like someone was really interested in me. She promised she would take good care of me, and I believed her. It has now been ten years and I still see her regularly, just to get my "six month warranty renewed!" She is always there for me, and I am at peace that she has my best interest at heart. I was so lucky to find her.

I was pretty much an emotional mess during all the treatment and needed a distraction. I decided to write a program for physical therapists about rehabilitating total knee patients. That was always my passion, and I needed an outlet. So, at night, I would escape (literally and figuratively) to the guesthouse and start writing. My girls were having a hard time at sixteen and seventeen, but I couldn't deal with it myself much less with them. So I continued to run and hide.

During radiation, I met a fellow therapist about ten years older than myself and we became "Wine and Whine" buddies. The support groups were so depressing we couldn't stand it, so we supported each other. Once a week we would meet and discuss our fears, problems and concerns (basically a bitch session!) and spare our spouses and families. Now that was therapeutic!

In July of that same year, my children's stepmother was also diagnosed with breast cancer. She was 35 years old with a family history, and thus had bilateral mastectomies and reconstruction. We were all shocked. This cancer thing was all around us. My girls were really getting nervous, and I was not sure how much that family talked about it either.

Then, three months later, after a much-needed time out just with Bob, Dad phoned with another bombshell. Mom had breast cancer. I was numb. This was unbelievable. My children's step mom, grandmother and I all had breast cancer within a nine month time frame. My poor girls, now at seventeen and eighteen, were feeling the curse.

My sisters and I all rallied to Mom's side, and I must admit now, I was pretty useless. The pain of reliving all that over again, and the thought of Mom going through the mental and physical pain was overwhelming. So, once again, I blocked it out of my mind. The only thing I was good at was keeping Dad company having a "toddy for the body" with him on the porch. Mom was so strong and amazing through it all, and she did great.

I had learned a thing or two, and so when I finally became conscious again, I shared with her some important facts. Actually, after talking to Mom, and Miss Yvonne (our Michigan friend who also had breast cancer that summer) I decided to try and find some humor in this very sensitive subject. So, I wrote "A Therapist's Tips for Treating the Tittie". It pretty much outlined all aspects of surviving the lumpectomy and radiation and added a little humor to lift the soul at the same time. I have since shared this with my surgeon and many other friends who were unfortunate enough to need it! (I have added it to the back of this book along with Larry's Laws For The Loveless, just in case someone else needs it too. Remember, be prepared!)

By school time, I was finally able to deal with all the cancer stuff, but noticed that Steve was having a hard time. He would cry and hang onto my leg before kindergarten, and that just broke my heart. The girls were not getting along then either, and Ed became very quiet. I felt my family falling apart, but I was now strong enough to ask for help.

Nobody liked admitting that you need help, but when you finally are being helped it is a Godsend. I took three months off work, and we began weekly family therapy. We all hated it, but somebody needed to get us all talking. Our family had been through so much: a new marriage, death of a baby, new baby, breast cancer for Mom and family, and we wondered why we were all so stressed? Within a few months the weight was lifted, and we could get on with our lives. Almost gone…

I survived breast cancer, and my third life would start.

15

Slow Down and Smell the Roses!

People respond differently to life and death experiences. For me, I know it was a blessing. It made Bob and me put our life into perspective. Being married with four children, we were always running. Playing tag team and running.

Working, and running. Always running to school, practice or some event. Running ourselves ragged! Cancer was our gift. We finally slowed down. We realized that things do work out for the best.

We no longer live for tomorrow, we embrace today. I love my job, but I love my kids more. I realized that even in middle and high school, even though they say only a few words, they like you around.

I always said that some of my goals were to travel, to rock babies and to learn Spanish. I made time for two out of three. I began working only one day a week. I worked on my Home Study course from home, and eventually even dissolved my little company I started after my breast cancer. My girls were off to college, and I loved being the "consultant" now. I am so proud of them and enjoy being with their friends. The boys are so easy, feed them and watch plenty of sports. I am good at that.

So, I took the first step towards my goals and went to Parkland Hospital to volunteer. This is an experience in itself! The place is huge. I managed to find the Volunteer office and met the most outgoing female on the planet.

She talked faster than I did! She was my age, single, no kids and worked like a Trojan. She had been there for at least twenty years and knew EVERYTHING about Parkland. We became instant friends. That day she reviewed my shot record and I was good to go. She grabbed another volunteer as we were walking up to the baby floor and introduced us and then said, "She'll tell you what to do, she is the best!" She was. I admitted my fears about this entire adventure, and then June told me her story. She lost her baby to SIDS many years ago and had begun volunteering as "her therapy". I told her about my baby, and said I didn't think the NNICU was for me. "OH, yes, it is! WE need you desperately! Do you realize that this hospital delivers 16,000 babies a year? Those other babies usually have Mom's to come see them, our babies usually don't." She took my hand and led me into the unit. "Let's go."

We walked into the first room and there were five little incubators, called isolettes on each side of the room, with these teeny babies all hooked up to monitors, and machines. I took one look and said, "June, I'm not sure I can do this."

My hands began to shake and as I peeked into the incubators, tears formed in my eyes. They were so tiny! Just like Scott! How could I do this? I really just wanted a little hugging therapy, to cuddle with some cute, fat little healthy babies. These were so fragile! I fought back the tears. This was going to be challenging.

She brought me over to the first nurse and introduced me. "Would you like to feed this baby?" she asked. "Me? This is my first day, and I am a serious rookie." "Don't you have children? You will do fine." She handed me this little bundle all wrapped up tight like a burrito, and the smallest bottle I'd ever seen. It only had about 30 ml, which is about one oz of formula. My little Steve weighed in at almost nine pounds and he was sucking down at least eight times that much. I'd never seen such a small baby or bottle. We both did fine, and I even managed not to get all the wires tangled up. The first week I came home with such a horrific neck ache, and upon analyzing my positions realized that I was all hunched over holding onto those little bundles so tight. I was so afraid to drop one.

After about a year, I relaxed a little. I learned what all the machines did and what was normal and abnormal. But, not without a few memorable moments.

Those nurses just amaze me. Each baby has its own set of bells for different problems, and at any given moment there are at least two babies bells ringing signaling decreased blood oxygen levels, heart rate abnormalities, medicines, and nasal cannulas for oxygen. Sometimes it is non stop! The stress is UNBELIEVABLE! At first I would go home and be so hyped up and stressed out that my family questioned why I was doing this. "I like it, and they need me so badly" was my response.

I'm much better now. I love those little ones that weigh about three pounds have a head the size of your fist and are so alert and cute. I had a little one yesterday that was so tiny but was alert. I looked and sure enough, she had been born seven months earlier, at 28 weeks! She was the cutest little thing, three pounds and had just gotten off the oxygen. I can't even imagine having a baby stay in the hospital that long, but they do. Sometimes I get so sad. I have seen so many different problems and so many "babies having babies". Some days are very hard to deal with. Life and death of an infant. I am so thankful that I have the opportunity to give a little bit of loving to these precious little angels.

Traveling was my next goal. Bob, being self employed, was always hesitant to leave town for longer than three days. Our usual routine included our official Saturday date night, and Friday night Mexican dinner with the kids. But after our "wake up call" we started taking a long vacation. We both wanted to visit Europe and so we did. Every two years since my cancer, we take a ten-day vacation, just the two of us.

The first trip to Europe was quite eventful. Bob and I were so excited. He didn't close his eyes the entire trip and by the time we arrived in Paris he was exhausted. But, we kept moving. We had arranged to meet some Italian friends of mine that day.

I met Dianno and Elisabeta fifteen years earlier when they were briefly in Dallas for business, and we became fast friends. They flew in to meet Bob and me and to spend the weekend with us in Paris. It was a scene right out of a movie when we met up with them. Walking down Rue. St. Michel after our café au lait, I glanced up and there she was. I took another look to be sure, and she spotted me. Within seconds, with stretched out arms we were running towards each other through the maze of pedestrians. Running and screaming we finally embraced! We hugged and cried and began talking so fast in English and Italian! Our two husbands who had never met before just stared at each other. After many minutes of crying, kissing and hugging, I introduced Bob to Dianno. They became instant friends (neither one spoke much) and it didn't hurt that they were both civil engineers. Elisabeta's English was a little rusty and my Spanish/Italian was even worse, but we were so happy to be together again.

We celebrated and had two great days touring the City of Lights. We had a so much fun, eating escargot and all the other fabulous dishes, drinking lots of wonderful wine, and cruising down the Seine. We all hated to see the weekend end, and promised not to wait fifteen more years to get together. (We kept our promise and met them in Rome four years later!) AH…Life is good!

A few days later, the excitement began. Now having the time to ourselves that is so rare and precious in our home, I decided to add to this romantic city a romantic moment. Anyone who knows me should already be laughing for I can never pull off anything like that. Anyway, I gave a new meaning to the phase "Come on baby light my fire!"

Our hotel room was matchbox small, but we had a great little pink marble bathroom with a Jacuzzi tub. (It was small too!) I brought along a few candles, just in case, and so I set the stage with the candles and a little wine. No sooner had I closed my eyes and eased under the water to relax when I smelled something burning. Oh no, it can't be! I screamed, bolted from the tub, grabbed a towel and frantically started swatting the fire that the candle had started with the toilet paper! Bob walked in, sees me standing in the buff, madly slinging the towel at the fire in a smoky bathroom and in his sarcastic Michigan voice said, "What are you doing?" I replied in my calmest voice, "I was just preparing for a romantic moment!" He shakes his head and replied "Next time, can you try not to burn down the hotel during this romantic moment! They don't even have a sprinkler system!" A sprinkler system! Can you believe he would actually think about that? Only an engineer would have noticed that small detail. So much for romance with a Yankee engineer!

We had a great trip to France and met so many wonderful people. It is amazing how many other couples we met who had experienced serious trauma and also made major life changes. I am a slow learner, but I do learn. I know how fragile life is, and I do believe everyday is a gift.

Midway through our trip, we drove from Paris and stayed in a few Relais and Chateau's. Bob was a bit nervous driving on the motorways and through all the tunnels, but he did fine. Mom gave us all the information, and we selected a couple of relais south-east of Paris. They were beautiful. We arrived at the second one situated on the south side of Lake Geneva. It was so old! It was an old castle and had three floors and a gorgeous view of the lake. We checked in and upon receipt of the brass key were immediately told, "You have the smallest room in the castle." We laughed. Remembering how much the smallest room cost, I couldn't imagine what the largest cost.

On our second day we decided to go across the Lake to Lausanne, Switzerland by ferry. We drove to Evian (the water place), to pick up the boat. As we were driving down this beautiful, waterfront two lane road, Bob quietly announced that was having a spell. "What?" I frantically screamed.

"I'm having a spell." he said. "Like your heart spell?" I inquired.

"Yes" he says. "Pull Over! Pull Over!" I yell over and over. He just kept driving. What seemed like hours later (it was probably seconds) he finally pulled into a parking lot. I checked his pulse and it was 250 beats per minute! "Oh my God, it's 250!" I screamed. "What do you want me to do?"

This was not the first "spell" for Bob. He had begun having them years earlier, and all the trips to the ER had been in vain since no one ever got an EKG strip with the abnormality on it. He had been "spell free" for over a year, but naturally, on our first trip across the pond, he had one! After a minute or so, I took charge. "Let's go to the hospital." Of course we have absolutely NO idea where a hospital is in this quaint little town in France!

I ran from the car and began searching for someone...anyone who could help me. I finally located a gentleman and in my best French screamed, "Where is a hospital?" The fellow must have seen the urgency on my face and he rattled off something with accompanying hand gestures. I took off. Bob was lying down in the back seat and I jumped in the driver's spot. I turned the key and prepared to accelerate and noticed it was a stick shift car. I hadn't driven a car like this since my brother-in-law Wendell taught me 25 years earlier. I shifted and clutched and we eased forward, then bucked back and forth, but finally took off. I didn't know I was going down a one way street the wrong way, but we made it to the main drag. My angels were watching again for at the next intersection I saw the big H sign and turned left. We were two blocks from the hospital!

I parked the car and took off running to the entrance. Then I came back and walked with Bob. We reached the admitting area and not knowing enough French I started beating my chest and screaming, "CARDIO, CARDIO." The nurse grabbed me and started to take ME back, when I shouted, "No not me, HIM!" They took Bob back and immediately began hooking him up to the machines. This heart episode of tachycardia lasted about thirty minutes, so the doctors were able to get the EKG we needed. It was mid afternoon by the time things settled down and although we had the number of the cardiologist at UT Southwestern, we felt like he was in good hands here.

I can't say enough about the care we received. First of all, he was taken in and his treatment began LONG BEFORE any paperwork was generated. Even through only one nurse spoke English, we were informed of every test result. A cardiologist was consulted, and after about four hours we were discharged. We left the ER with prescriptions, and directions to the pharmacy, and headed for the cashier window. We inquired about the bill, and they said we didn't owe anything, they would send us a bill. Do you believe this? Four hours of great emergency room treatment, with every test known to mankind, a fabulous lunch and we didn't have to pay a dime. We finally got a bill two months later for $200. Now I am really convinced our medical system needs work.

Bob was exhausted when we got back to the castle. He went to lie down, and I digested the instructions. No more traveling by car, as Bob could not drive at all. (This news almost sent him into another tizzy, the thought of me driving him around in Europe.) Mom always said the concierges at all the hotels can take care of anything, so I marched off to find ours. We needed to stay at the castle for the remainder of our trip, cancel other reservations, return the car, and somehow get back to Paris!

I found our concierge, and upon relaying the day's events, I fell apart. I was so worried about Bob and the fact that I might have lost him. So as I was hysterically crying, the concierge assured me he would take care of everything. And he did. He was terrific. We stayed in the "smallest room" for four more days and really enjoyed it. Bob was afraid to drink, so I had my share and his share! I do love French wines!

We made it home safely and Bob had his heart procedure not long after. Everything went well. Things do work out for the best!

During the next few months, I was healing emotionally, and physically from the cancer trauma, but I needed to heal spiritually. My friend Karen was my inspiration. A year after my cancer, Karen's breast cancer came back with a vengeance. It had metastasised to her lungs between her annual checkups. She was six years out from her first episode and now she started the battle again. More chemotherapy, more hair loss, more pain and yet, she never gave up hope. She had such faith in God, courage and strength. She invited me to her healing service one morning.

Karen was a Baptist, I'm a Catholic and the service was at an Episcopal Church. It was fantastic. Every week we would go with about forty older people, all there to pray for healing of one kind or another. It was absolutely the most spiritual, uplifting experience. Each week we talked about death and the after life, and before too long, I finally came to some peace about dying. It was wonderful. I would cry knowing about Karen's suffering and her fate, but she never did. She was so brave and so strong. I learned about true courage from Karen.

My Dad was always telling me to slow down and smell the roses, and I finally have. I walk almost everyday, and I enjoy the clouds, the sky and the flowers so much more now. I try to find something fun in life everyday, and somehow this seems to be getting easier!

16

Finding Fun at Fifty!

Five years ago, I hit a milestone birthday, the big 50. I wasn't so sure "fifty was nifty," but Sue and the family were going to do their best to make it fun.

On the Friday of St. Patrick's Day weekend, my daughter Liz was home from college, and she greeted me with a cup of coffee as I walked out of the bedroom. This should have been my first clue, that this day was going to be different, but I missed it. She then asked if she could walk with me. So I donned my *Race for the Cure* T shirt, sweat pants and tennis shoes, and we were out the door.

After circling the block, Liz then proceeded to say, "Sorry Mom, but I have to do this" and she blindfolded me. Well, I started laughing and said, "OK what's going on?" We walked a few more feet and then she said, "Now get in. Duck your head." I was laughing so hard and then I heard more giggles coming from the front seat. "Who is there?" No answer, but another chuckle. I started flinging my arms and felt long hair, and so I guessed, "Char, is that you?" Then another giggle and I heard my niece Katherine.

"What is going on here?" Liz had placed a tiara on my head, and all the girls were laughing.

My wonderful sister Sue had arranged for this kidnapping for my birthday. We were all headed to Jackson, Mississippi to march in the St. Patrick's Day Parade. I screamed with excitement. "Are we really marching? What will we wear?" I had no purse, no money, and no clothes! Sue had set this weekend up with all the loved ones in my life that she knew could handle such fun. Charlotte, Liz, Bob and Katherine had all worked together to pull it off. Liz had packed my clothes, Char had reading material for the car trip, Katherine brought tiaras, and Sue had Mom, Dad, Rosie (our adopted sister) and friend Angie meeting us in Jackson. Bob knew this was going to be a wild and crazy weekend, so he politely offered to stay home with the boys and animals. This was going to be a memorable birthday for sure.

This trip was planned after Sue and I finished what has to be an all time favorite book. Jill Conner Browne from Jackson, Mississippi, wrote the book _The Sweet Potato Queens_ _Book of Love,_ absolutely the funniest book I have ever read! Since my repertoire of reading material has been narrowed down to "Smut Books" ("Lovie books" as my son calls them) and books that make you laugh, this one hit the spot.

Jill, THE Boss Queen of her group of friends (The Sweet Potato Queens) decided to march in the parade about twenty years ago. Well, her books (she now has five of them, and I suggest you run, not walk to the nearest book store to pick them up) have made it to the "big time" (New York Times Best Seller list). She has empowered women to take some time off and be Queenly! Boas and tiaras mandatory! She also lets everyone march in the parade with her! Women from all over the nation come for this special weekend and dress up and play.

We all know that life and motherhood can be so exhausting, stressful and over-whelming that women today are basically burned out. Jill's books are an outlet for fun and laughter, and if you are lucky enough to make it to Jackson for the St. Paddy's Day parade, you will seriously get your battery re-charged! It is really Spring Break for Moms, and the most fun weekend (without your spouses) ever.

The Friday night activities started in our hotel room. Mom and Dad brought crawfish and snacks, and we had more booze than a bootlegger! So the partying started! My birthday gifts were opened, official Sweet Potato Queen sunglasses, long gloves, and new boas along with my new threads from the girls. After a few cocktails, we were all so excited that Mom was jumping on the bed with Sue! Now Mom is the spryest 70ish-year-old you have ever seen, and she also likes to have a good time.

We headed out to the meeting place, Hal and Mal's establishment with the other 500 + fun seeking women. There was great music, food and of course more tod-dies. We all had a ball. After a few hours, the Queens appeared and they were just darling! I had been "over served" and was on my way to La La land when I was introduced to the Boss Queen, Jill. Seems I was hanging all over the poor woman, in my condition, but she was a sport and just was as gracious as could be. It was too much fun, dancing and carrying on. We started back for the hotel on foot, and got lost. The fine law enforcement of Jackson saw this group of degenerates, figured we were harmless, and kindly put us on the right path toward the hotel. What a night!

So there we were, Texas clan and the Bay folks. Liz picked out old Prom dresses for herself and me, Katherine and Sue went "formal shopping" at the local Thrift store and the rest decided to be spectators.

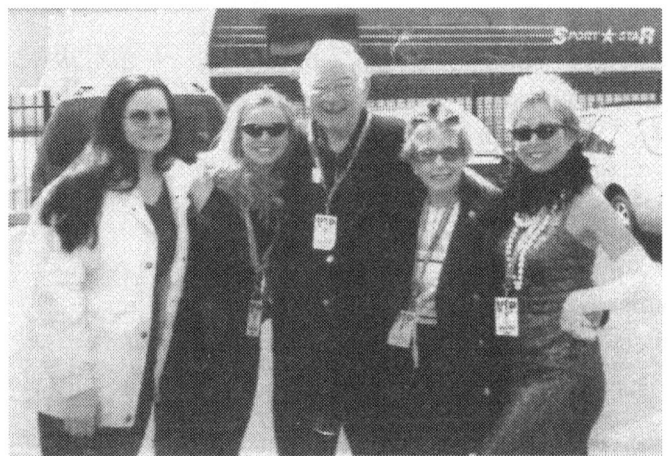

Charlotte, Liz, Potsy, Momsy, and I ready to go to the parade

The next morning, still fuzzy from the night before, I meandered down for some coffee and saw all these women dressed up! They had all sorts of outfits on, from prisoner's outfits, to Cotton queens to Krispy Queens. They were a hoot! I rallied immediately and asked why they were dressed so early. They informed me that we needed to be lining up to parade at 10:00. No, not 10! My group was still sleeping! So off I went. I was on a mission. Woke up the girls, jumped in the shower and donned my royal blue sparkly sequined formal with gloves, boa, tiara, and tennis shoes and knocked on Mom and Dad's door.

Mom slowly opened the door, saw me in my outfit, and just screamed, "OH Gary, You HAVE to come see Carol!" "What's wrong? Don't you like my outfit?" She was laughing so hard I thought she would fall on the floor. I nabbed three Advil and went back to the girls' room. Mom decided to pass on marching with us. (Could she have been embarrassed to be with me?)

We all finally got ready and although it was pretty cold, I decided to forgo the coat. Why lose the look? We all gathered for a hardy breakfast, and I wish you could have seen the people's faces when we walked into that restaurant all dressed for parading. People were laughing and staring. We just gave our queenly wave and told them to come to the parade.

Then we made one last trip back to the room for refreshments. As we walked into the hotel, a cute young woman with two teenage girls was checking in. She took one look at us and exclaimed, "I wanted to do that. Are ya'll marching in the Parade?" "We are, why aren't you?" She explained that she could not find anyone to go with her, so she was here to buy prom dresses for her girls. "No problem honey," I said. "We have an extra dress and I think it will fit you, come on." She passed keys and a credit card to the daughter, and off she went. "By the way, what's your name?" I asked. "Margo, from Chatham." We met our new best friend, Margo, right then. My angels were working again.

As luck would have it, the dress fit Margo like a glove, a lovely, purple sparkly number. She looked smashing! This was one of those moments that reinforces that there is a God who takes care of us. Meeting Margo was meant to be.

Sue and Margo were walking together to the parade route, yapping along and Sue gave her my story and that this was my birthday surprise. Then Margo told Sue her story. She had been through some tough times.

Three years ago, her husband left her with three kids. Two years ago, in March, she was diagnosed with a brain tumor and underwent surgery. Last year she said she was so depressed she cried the entire day. This year she screamed, "I met ya'll and I'm marching in the Sweet Potato Queens Parade! This is so much fun! Thank ya'll!" And it was. She is a special lady and we love her.

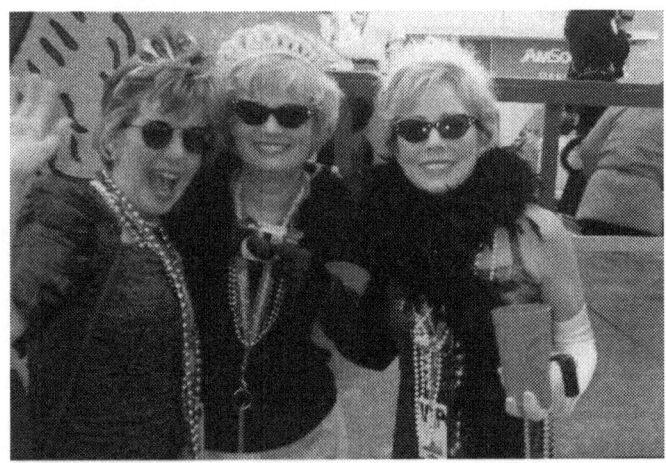

Margo, Sue, and me

We watched the people gather round and were just shocked. There were so many people! Woman of all ages, all sizes and shapes, dressed in "queenly attire" and having fun. We heard later there were 2,000 marchers in the parade that year. And 60,000 spectators! Why go to Mardi Gras when you can have so much more fun here? I just hope we can keep the secret!

So the five of us with no beads to throw, no nothing, simple rookies, just commenced waving and smiling. We marched behind the Teenie Weenie Bikini Queenies from South Carolina and they were a riot. We were all in our forties and fifties and they were closer to sixty, seventy range. They wore T-shirts with bikinis outlined on them and sang a song that said they were looking for a "Big, fat weenie!" We were appalled! But we died laughing! They found out we had wine and they were our new best friends! Then we found out (they flashed us) they actually wore thongs under the T-shirts! We were so grossed out! It was definitely an experience!

After marching we went back to Hal and Mal's for more partying. Now we had the cutest young girls in the world with us, our daughters, so it didn't take us long to hook up with all sorts of precious guys in their mid 20's and 30's trying hard to make points with the mamas to get to the girls. Oh, Southern boys are so smart! They knew this parade weekend was a harvesting ground for women so the local men came out to play too. They bought us drinks and gave us beads and even started calling me "Mother in law!" They were darling. The "Bo Peeps" (the nickname for the daughters of Queens) had a great time too. Why don't the guys in Texas act like this, I wondered?

Then Sue and I wandered around and found the back porch to this huge place. Low and behold, we found THE REAL QUEENS! There they were, in the flesh, just having a good time like everybody else. Naturally we made quite a scene like they were indeed royalty or movie stars. We met Jill, the Boss Queen, who forgave me for hanging all over her the previous evening, and Donna and her boyfriend. We shared the birthday surprise/kidnapping story with them and they loved it. Since I had worked in Jackson many moons ago, I started the "do you know" game and sure enough she did know my friend. Tammy Donna was my instant new best friend. She was actually the nicest, cutest person, just a regular Mom like the rest of us. It was so much fun!

Since that first year, we have been back six more times. The Margarita Mammas were officially inaugurated the following year, and I was chosen Boss Queen of our group. We had 21 members, Queens, Bo Peeps, Wannabees and Spud Studs, and last year we went all out with "exotic dance wear" as our dress for the parade with 31 members! I am trying to keep this a select group, but with Sue inviting everybody (because she is like that) it is very difficult. No doubt though, that first year had to have been the best birthday I had ever had. This new decade was looking good so far!

17

The End of Our World

For me, I always have to have some fun, because before you can blink an eye, you will be required to be strong again. Fun and sun recharge my battery for the next crisis.

A few months later was Dad's 80th birthday and the Texas families decided to celebrate in our favorite place, Cozumel, Mexico. We gathered all the college kids, and Ed and Steve and took off for an unforgettable Easter weekend. Three days of sunning, snorkeling, eating and playing together. There is nothing better.

Sue had organized a Birthday "Book" and had all of the families and friends send pictures and stories of special times with Dad. It was a scrapbook of his life that was so special. The stories were so heart warming; before dinner was over we were all in tears. He is truly an incredible man. His professional life was the epitome of the American dream, work hard and rise to the top. He began his career as a salesman, and retired as the President and CEO of a large company. He had numerous friends, a warm, loving family life, and he was without a doubt, the most optimistic person on this earth. Mom was so proud. We were so blessed, he and Mom were healthy and active, and they had been together 58 years! We knew we were lucky and hoped we had lots of good years ahead. We had a wonderful family and we all were so grateful.

September 11, 2001 rocked all of our worlds. Freedom was no longer to be taken for granted, and terrorism was a reality. I feared for my two brothers, one in Washington and the other traveling internationally. They both came home safely, but we all still worried and remained on high alert.

Two months later, I was planning Thanksgiving at our new home. Mom and Dad, Sue's family and Dean's family were all going to be together for the first time. I was thrilled. Cooking and planning were all part of the fun. I could finally use that big table we had bought just for this type of occasion. I was preparing for the family when I got a call from my sister-in-law Marilene the Sunday before Thanksgiving. She was worried about my Mom, saying she was a little forgetful, and felt she should have a checkup before coming to Dallas. (I had no problem with this since three years earlier we ended up taking Mrs. Lander to the emergency room with a blood pressure problem.)

I called Dad and talked to him and he didn't seem too worried. He agreed to take her in to see the doctor and assured me they would make the flight on Wednesday. Monday night, Dad called and said the doctors wanted to run some tests at the hospital the next day, and he would keep me posted. He felt like maybe this had been a little mini stroke, but nothing too serious.

Dean's family arrived the next evening after a long, hard ten hour drive with their three kids! We gathered at Sue and Wade's restaurant ready to begin the celebration. After all the hugs and kisses, Sue pulled me aside and told me Dad had just called and they still didn't know what was wrong with Mom, but they were still coming. The doctors were thinking it was the beginning of Alzheimer's disease. We were all dazed and tried to look on the bright side. I was upset, and Bob tried to cheer me up by saying, "Be thankful, it could be worse. It's not a brain tumor." That did help a little.

The next morning, bright and early, Marilene and I took off for our walk. It was nice to get a chance to catch up on all the family gossip! With four brothers and sisters, twenty grandchildren and two great grandchildren in the family we had lots to talk about. We got home at about ten, and the phone was ringing. It was Sue. REAL Bad News…it WAS a brain tumor! My medical brain kicked into gear and I yelled, "How can they change their diagnosis from Alzheimer's to a brain tumor over night?" Sue was hysterical. Dean walked in the house just in time to hear the conversation, and within seconds was on his cell phone. I called my pathologist friend at the local hospital and asked him to go see Mom and read her chart. He called me back a few minutes later and confirmed the diagnosis, brain cancer called glioblastoma multiformae.

"Carol, it's big, and in-operable." I remembered just enough about neuropathology to recall that this was the absolute worse kind of brain cancer and that it was very aggressive. "Phil what do I do? Should we all come home now or should we wait a few days?" He thought we should come home immediately. I was sick. I knew what that meant. Not Mom. Oh God help us! I am not sure we can survive without her.

Dean's family had not even unpacked yet so they were back on the road. I was in shock, so Bob took over. Sue's family was flying out on an afternoon flight, and Ed made me a reservation on the same plane. Liz and her dog come in from college, and were told not to unpack; they were driving to the Bay. I got a few things together and left for the airport.

I met Sue's family at the airport and we all started crying. "This can't be happening to Mom! She is so healthy! She had survived breast cancer and a few skin cancers and was in great shape. She just drove Dad to Atlanta and back two weeks ago. She had no symptoms, how can this be?" We were all devastated. No one spoke and everyone cried. We had no idea what to do.

The family rallied together for one last Thanksgiving together. Everyone came in from all over. Mom was discharged on the day after Thanksgiving so we had dinner that day. It was a bittersweet day.

The family supported Dad as best we could. The girls took turns staying a week at a time, and the boys were there daily. We lost her six weeks later.

I was lucky enough to be with her for the last week. She went to a party at the Yacht Club on Saturday, then we had a Mass at the house on Sunday. Dean took us all to dinner for New Year's Eve, and we went to his house on New Year's Day. She saw the doctor the next day, and I left on Thursday to go back to Dallas. Before I left early the next morning, I tiptoed in her room and kissed her goodbye. "I'll be back, and I love you".

"I know you do," she replied. That was the last thing I said to her. Mom had a major seizure the next day after lunch and was gone.

There are no words to describe the loss of your best friend, your Mom. She was without a doubt the nucleus of our family. She was so loving and caring, always giving to her friends and family, many times until she was physically exhausted and ill. She was a gracious lady, a class act. After Uncle Henry died, I was on Dean's boat with the family spreading his ashes and crying so hard. I don't know why I chose that time, (probably cause she took care of Henry too) but I told her how great we thought she was and that none of us could ever measure up to her no matter how hard we tried. It was the truth.

She was so special to all of us in different ways. She supported me through all of my crises, she was there for all the grandchildren, she was the backbone for Gene's political career, and she had such a special relationship with Di and Sue. She even managed to stay friends with two out of three out laws!

The night she died, when I was back at the house with Dad, during the local 10 o'clock news, they announced her passing. I was so surprised, yet, after a few minutes, I realized it was so fitting. She had so many friends and had been such a loving "Momsy" to so many that she deserved "a celebrity's" farewell.

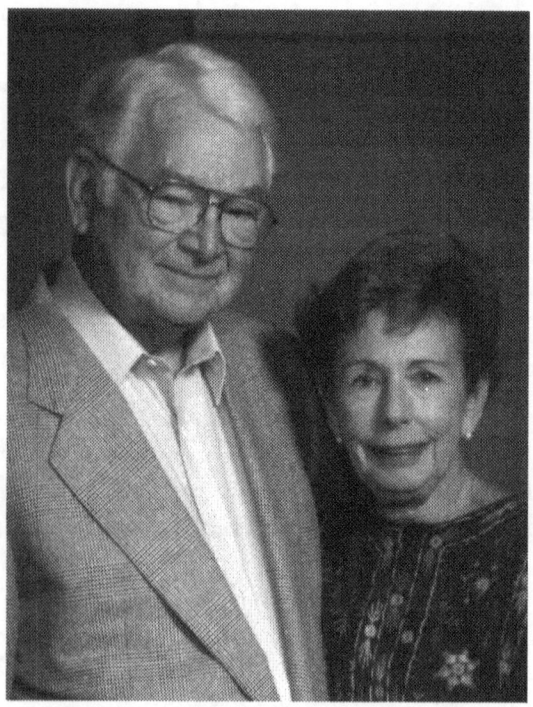

Mom and Dad married 58 years

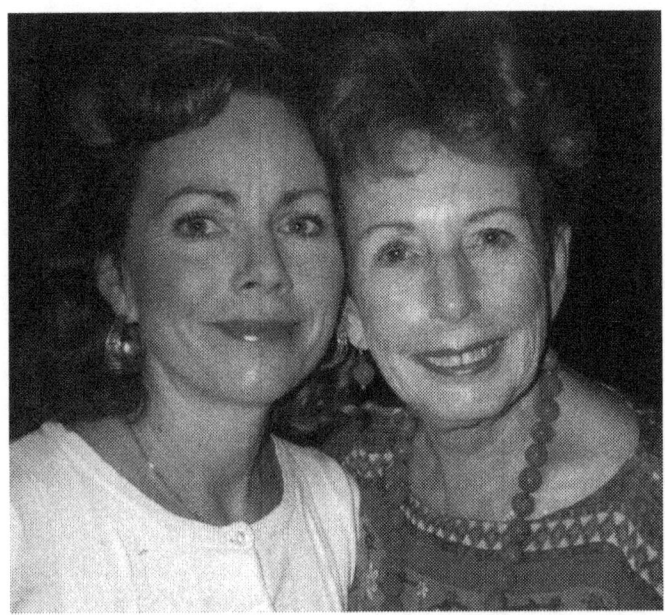

Mom and I celebrating in Mexico the year we both had breast cancer, 1996

Healing takes time, and I am not there yet. I miss her so much, and I talk to her regularly during my walks. Sometimes, I just wish she would talk louder! Then I know, I need to slow down, be quiet and listen. She is now our angel, at peace and safely home in that heavenly country with Don, Nana and her Dad, rocking my baby Scott, and Di's baby, and taking care of all those "old coots" that have gone before Dad. She may be gone, but she is certainly not forgotten.

18

Still Vertical and Coping with Cancer

Mom's death was so traumatic for all of us, and I learned that people grieve and heal differently. My mind and body were slowly healing but I needed a diversion.

Then, fortunately came St. Paddy's weekend in Jackson and we had a mission. Last year, Mom and Dad both came and Dad had such a good time that we thought this would be a great escape for him. So, Sue called and he and Rosie agreed to meet us in Jackson.

The Dallas/Denton girl friends had all seen the pictures and were all begging to be admitted into the group. As "Boss Queen" I had a little bit of say in this process, but not much. So, before you could blink an eye, we had 21 members of the Margarita Mamas! Costumes were decided upon, sarongs with white shirts, boas, and crowns and we were set. Since a few Spud Studs (husbands who were roped into helping out) had decided to join the group, we ordered a banner for them to carry with our official group name. Margo kept in touch throughout the year via email and she met us there. Friday afternoon came and we all descended upon the hotel. We had rooms on the pool floor and proceeded to "take over the place". Dad and Rosie came and he looked good. He needed a weekend away. He had a good time the first year, but as a single Spud, the second year, in a party that is 99% females, he REALLY had fun.

It did us all good to play again. We were still hurting from losing Mom, and it felt good to laugh and have a little fun. Good fun is a pre-requisite for recharging my battery, and I definitely needed a jumpstart! Everyday is a gift and you just never know about tomorrow.

A few months later, I had another scare. A lump on my other breast appeared. The birthday biopsy (the only day the surgeon could do it) was negative and I had dodged another bullet. Thank the Lord.

Aging is the pits, so many things to keep looking out for. Then one day I noticed an "age spot" on my face that had developed a mole in it. I watched it for a few months, and it got darker. With Mom's history of basal cell carcinoma, and since I had one removed many years earlier, I decided to have it checked.

I went in to the dermatologist in July, since I was taking the kids to Mexico for a few days. Waiting in the doctor's office, I picked up the brochure on skin cancers. "I had a basal cell taken off my neck a long time ago, but this looks different" I said to the nurse. Yes, it did. Then I saw it. The other picture on the brochure looked exactly like my mole, and it said Melanoma under it! "Does this look to you like what I have?" I asked the nurse. She looked at the picture, my face, the picture and said, "It sure does!" AHHH!! I freaked. I couldn't just have the "ordinary" basal cell, just my luck I would have the mega monster of all skin cancers, the kind that CAN KILL you! The doctor arrived and looked it over and very calmly stated that we would do a biopsy. "It's probably OK, but we want to be sure" he said. Mom had basal cell carcinomas for years and preached sunscreen to all of us light-eyed kids, but we didn't take her too seriously. Anyway, I needed the sun to recharge my battery!

I couldn't believe it. The week I was to leave for a trip to Mexico with the kids, I got the phone call at work. "Hi, it's Dr. H. I can't believe it, but your biopsy came back positive for melanoma." Pause. Oh, no, not again. It was the big mother of skin cancers.

"Am I going to die?" I asked the doctor. "Probably not, but you need to see the surgeon as soon as you can" was his answer. Here we go again.

I took the kids to Mexico anyway, and was very sun cautious, even though I was still ignorant of the severity of the situation. I really needed my snorkeling! It is my therapy.

Floating in that beautiful crystal clear, turquoise blue water, gazing at the amazing world beneath the ocean with the most brilliantly colored fish, just gliding through the water, kissing the sand every so often, and swimming away is the most peaceful experience for me. So quiet, so beautiful, so serene. I treasure my time snorkeling.

It took me a couple of weeks to get the surgical teams' schedules together.

This small spot on my right cheek was going to require a Mohs specialist and a plastic surgeon. Sue and I went in for the first consult and I was given the ten-page booklet on the stages of melanoma and treatment approaches. She took notes for Bob. Seems my lesion was initially diagnosed to be .5mm deep. At 1.0 mm all hell breaks loose, and not just figuratively. Chemotherapy and other unpleasant treatments are needed. But I was lucky once again.

I saw the plastic surgeon and tried to be upbeat about all this. I even tried to negotiate a deal. "You're going to put one big scar on this side, so how about taking two big wrinkles off this side?" He wasn't amused. "This is serious, Carol. It will be a long scar down the entire length of your cheek, and it will take about a year to heal." "Great. OK, let's go" I said.

Bob had been through this so many times with me, and he and Sue now have a system. She brings me for the first phase, and Bob comes later. So, I went in and they drew a purple ring around my mole the size of the initial cut. This was a pretty big circle. Even Bob was shocked at the extent of the cut. After microscopic examination, if all the borders are clear of cancer cells, a bandage would be placed over the area, and I'd be sent to the hospital where the plastics doctor worked his magic to sew me up. I knew what to ask for when it came to anesthesia (the good stuff), so I was pumped and ready to go.

Two hours later I came out with this huge bandage on my face. I went home and lay down with the ice on my face as instructed. Steve was a bit shocked at the bandage, but I assured him it was OK.

A little later, Bob and Steve went out to get some ice cream and I took my first look in the mirror. "Oh my gosh, there is a baseball in my face!" I screamed. No one was home. I looked again. The whole side of my face was so swollen I couldn't open my eye all the way. This was DEFINITELY NOT NORMAL! I knew if I waited for Bob he would probably say, "It'll be all right, let's wait until morning" so I didn't wait. I raced to the phone where my instructions still lay, and called the doctor's number. The answering service asked if it was an emergency and I said yes. The doctor called me right back. "You think it's a hematoma?" he asked. "YES," I screamed "and a big one!"

"How soon can you get to the hospital?" "Can I wear my PJ's?"

"Sure." "Then ten minutes." "See you there. Just walk in and go downstairs, I'll have a nurse looking out for you."

The boys come home and I was up waiting to go. "What's the matter?"

"Look at my face! Something is SERIOUSLY wrong! I've already called the doctor and we need to go back to the hospital." Off we went. The doctor was waiting (thank goodness). He took one look at my face and said, "Oh, my goodness! I am so sorry but we will have to take you back into surgery. You have a hematoma (lay mans terms a bleeding blood vessel) and we need to go in there and clean it out, take care of the vessel, and put a drain in your face to ensure this won't happen again." "Let's go" I said.

This ordeal started at 9pm and at 1:30 am I headed for home. Steve went to the neighbor's house and Ed was with his Dad, so it was just Bob and I. Poor Bob, he had to go to work at the crack of dawn, so he called me every hour to be sure things were OK.

I was NOT a pretty sight! They had sutured me up with the skin on my cheek pilled up like a mountain, and with this tube in the incision exiting from the back of my ear into a little bag pinned to my PJ's. I scared myself I looked so bad!

My darling Steve came home and was my little "gofer" for the day. I assured him I was all right, just looked like scar face. Then Ed came in and saw me laying on the couch. "Hi, Mom." I rolled over and he stopped dead in his tracks. "Ah, what happened to you?" I reminded him of my melanoma surgery, and that I had a little complication that required another surgery. "Can I get you anything? How about a smoothie, can you eat a smoothie?" The cure-all in all college kids' minds is the smoothie. "That would be great, Ed". My precious eighteen year old, six foot two basketball player was indeed rattled for the first time. He frantically asked, "How about a movie? Why don't you watch a movie? I'll pick one out for you." He put in the movie "Hoosiers" a basketball movie! I was so touched I began crying. I had absolutely no desire to watch a movie, but Ed was sure that it would make me feel better. Those boys can be so dear! No wonder Mom's have such a special bond with them. They aren't always there for you like your girls, but when they are, they are so sincere it melts your heart!

This time, I knew I needed to talk to the kids about all this cancer and reassured them I was going to be OK. (I hope!)

In early April, way before the skin cancer episode, Bob and I had scheduled a trip to Hawaii for the fall when Ed left for school. Any mother of a senior in high school knows this is absolutely the hardest year of your life and if you do survive unscathed you need to treat yourself to a nice trip. We still had all summer to endure with this fabulous eighteen year old who was ready to be "footloose and fancy free!"

Then the melanoma monster hit. Naturally the doctors give you the old "live your life" speech so we decided to cautiously make the trip. Hats, sun screen, shade, more sun screen.

As you can see, my life teeter totters between "I Love Lucy's" fun, and General Hospital melodrama. Our Maui trip was no exception.

We were enjoying coffee early one morning on the balcony of our room at the fabulous Maui Grand Hyatt hotel. While enjoying the magnificent view of the ocean, and mountains, from 22 stories up in our designated white terry cloth robes, finally, recovering from the plane ride and just beginning to relax, I sat back and marveled at how fortunate we were to be able to have this beautiful scene. As I glanced back to look in the room I realized that the sliding glass door was ajar, and since I hate to waste energy, I quickly grabbed the door and slid it closed. Within an instant, there was a slight CLICK. Bob looked at me and said, "Did you hear that click?" "What click?" I replied. "Oh no" he gasped, "You didn't just lock us out did you?" Uh, oh! "But it couldn't possibly happen. I just slid the door closed."

Lucy, you are in trouble now! He jumped from the chair and tried to open the door. No luck. He pulled harder. No luck. About this time his brain reverted to engineer's survival mode and you could actually see the "wheels turning" in his head trying to figure out how we were going to get back in the room.

I started laughing at this point. He was almost panic stricken! "Don't worry, we'll get in," I said. "OK, how, smarty?" So I leaned over the rail to see if anyone on one side of us is awake. Empty. I go to the other side and lean over. Again, there was not a soul in sight. Bob began to really get nervous and started assessing our tools. Coffee cups, paper, white robes. Hum, I surely wasn't going to drop mine to use as a flag, and I don't think he was too keen on dropping his either, so we just looked at each other." Let's just try to relax and wait until someone comes walking down below us and then we'll just yell for help," I suggested. "I am not yelling to someone 22 floors below me for help." Typical male response. "You know I will" I said. So we waited. Not long after, a pool worker was dragging his cleaning material rather slowly and I had my prey. "Excuse me!" I screamed as loud as I could. "We're locked out! Can you get someone to help us?" He looked at me like I was crazy. Fortunately we were in Hawaii, not in a foreign country and they could understand English. After a few more yelling sessions to various people, we finally had someone come spring us from the balcony." In the future," the manager announced laughing," place one of your swim fins in the doorway to ensure this doesn't happen again." So much for trying to conserve energy and save the planet!

I reassured Bob, once again, that life with me would never be boring!

Things are looking good again. I am really lucky. At 55, I have had both shoulders operated on from working on people for thirty-two years, both boobs cut up, a large Dr. Evil scar on my right cheek, and I'm in the best shape of my life! (No gout and no hemorrhoids! A favorite saying from family friend Tommy Foley!)

Every three to six months, I have my cancer check ups and my body screened for melanoma. It has been almost four years since my melanoma surgery and I am once again waiting. Waiting to hear if this latest freckle taken off my leg is melanoma. It never ends once you have cancer. Every three to six months, you are back seeing the doctors, praying that you will once again be sparred. You never forget, but you live cautiously, trying not to let it consume your life.

My philosophy has always been, "Expect the worst and hope for the best." This seems strange to some, but as optimistic as I am, I also very much like to Be Prepared. I know the drill if it is cancer, and I can rearrange my schedule if need be. We do not know God's "master plan" and just have to adjust to the challenges that are given to us. I really believe this is just life, not adversity, but reality. Life is not easy and everybody has something to deal with. Frankly, I am so lucky. This latest mole was benign, a narrow escape!

19

The Final Lesson

I have learned many lessons throughout these years. I have survived death, divorce, and two cancers, and I will cope with whatever is sent my way. "Whatever doesn't kill you makes you stronger," Clarrie declares in the movie *Steel Magnolias.* I firmly believe this and I am a mighty strong little woman! My husband and my kids have also survived life-threatening incidents. There is a reason we are here and our angels are taking good care of us.

This year for my birthday, Charlotte's friend, Sunny, a very talented young artist, gave me a collage featuring Dallas minister Charles Swindoll's, reflection on attitude. I have it on my kitchen counter for all the family to see daily.

It basically says, "The longer I live, the more I realize the impact of attitude on life…. It is more important than the past, than education, than money, than circumstance, than failures, than successes, than what other people think or say or do. …The remarkable thing is that we have a CHOICE every day regarding the attitude we will embrace for that day."

"We cannot change the inevitable. …I am convinced, that life is 10% what happens to me and 90% how I react to it". I totally agree.

I initially wrote that I was lucky for the following reasons, and one of my patients, Pastor Mays, corrected me as I was talking one day. "You are not lucky, Carol, you are blessed." By George, he's right: I'm not lucky, I'm blessed!

I am blessed to have had such a wonderful childhood with such a warm and loving family and friends. I am blessed to have grown up in a family with strong faith, and to have met others who have helped me survive life's hurricanes. I am blessed that I learned these life lessons that have given me the strength I needed to help me through these traumas. I am blessed that I was able to live in the New Orleans area where you learn not to be too serious all of the time and to enjoy life. Mostly, I am blessed to have such a wonderful husband who has been my strength and who has made my new life worth living. As Charlotte says, "He saved us" and enabled us to be a real family again.

Without these values and people in my life, I am sure my attitude would be different.

Every morning I am thrilled to wake up and be vertical, even though I have finally come to some peace about the fact that one day I won't. I love my family and can't wait to watch them have their own families and be a grandmother. Nobody can ever replace "Momsy" but we will all remember her loving caring ways and do our best to emulate her. I have learned so much from all of these crises, and I truly believe things do work out for the best.

We all have angels that make such an impact on our lives and support us through these challenging times. Some are more visible than others.

Mom was one of my living angels, as well as my "adopted" Aunt Peggy. Both of these women were from a mold that cannot be replaced. Aunt Peggy was my other Mom, and now has to fill in. She is one of the last "true ladies" of the South, soft spoken, kind, generous, loving and so very caring. Her daughter Polly was my childhood best friend and we had so many great times together. I failed charm school, but I hope that I can learn from Mom and Aunt Peggy how to be a good mother and a little bit of a lady.

The nurses in the neonatal intensive care unit where I volunteer each week are so good. They work so hard and are kind, patient and caring for those tiny little miracles, and they have to deal with such stress. I love going and hugging on those precious babies, but watching those nurses at work is so inspirational. They are angels.

The minister and the little ladies at the Healing Service are also my angels. They have been so supportive of me for the past five years. We lost our Karen three years ago. She was only 54 and she was such a trooper. She battled breast cancer the second time, for four years, with 64 chemotherapy treatments. She was so brave. She had a passion for work, and she continued until the week before she died. Karen's death was the epitome of faith, courage and dignity. She taught me so much.

Finally, what would I have done without my family, my patients, my sister, Sue, and her husband, Wade, my husband, and my Dad? For all the hurricanes in my life, they have kept my boat afloat. They are my angels. They have taught me so many valuable lessons. My favorite is to always live, love, and laugh.

My friend Carolyn and I were talking on one of the girls' trips to Mexico, and she remarked, "You know if this plane went down and we died tomorrow, people would say, 'Oh, they were 50. They lived their life.'"

I don't think so. I hope my life is only half over. I still have a passion for life and a whole lot more living to do! The fifth decade of life has been called the "Age of Wisdom and Wit". I love it!

As a mother, I still worry a lot about my children and the future. Pastor Mays also reminded me that a strong foundation could withstand a lot of gale force winds. I know I have a strong foundation, and now I know how strong the family foundation is. They were put to the test with Hurricane Katrina.

On August 26, 2005 I had just helped my daughter Liz fulfill her dream and move to Boston to practice physical therapy. Leaving the airport on the way back to Dallas I hear about a hurricane heading towards New Orleans and the Gulf Coast. Not another one, I thought.

I was in Gulfport for Dennis, saw Cozumel right after Emily and now here we go again.

Excited about Liz's new place and anxious to tell everyone about it, I forgot about the news. Two mornings later, I watched the news again and was paralyzed by this hurricane's size. "Oh, my gosh, this is it!" I yell at Bob. We watched together as the weather reporters warned of the destruction of a category five storm and of the devastation it could cause New Orleans and the Gulf Coast.

I started calling the family. Dad was still going through cardiac rehab after his quintuple by-pass surgery in late June and his medications were not balanced yet. His next appointment was set for Monday, the day the storm was supposed to hit. He did not seem to be worried and rejected my offer to come stay with us in Dallas. "Your brother is here and he has a generator. I'll be fine there on the farm."

Next call was to my sister-in-law Marilene on the farm. Please bring the family and come stay with us, I plead. I was so scared, and I had a bad feeling about this. She assured me that their home is the "safe" place because it is inland, and has a well and a generator. "I am a little worried about the roof on this new house, if the winds are as high as expected," she admitted. But, "we are fine and will stay here with Potsy, and Gene's family." Then I called my other sister-in-law, Margaret. "Are you leaving your home? Please come up here and stay with us!" She assured me that Gene would NEVER leave the area and that they would be on the farm with the rest of the family.

Finally, I called Rosie. She is our family friend for over 30 years, and is more like a sister. She so graciously let us stay in her home while Dad was in intensive care. I knew she was really stubborn and would not evacuate easily. "Please Rosemary, leave and go to the farm. (I knew Dallas was out of the question). She actually sounded a little scared and assured me she was leaving soon. I was a wreck. My entire extended family in harms way. The Mississippians were all staying on the farm, and Dianne and her family were in Baton Rouge. Although we thought they were safer, they were still at risk.

I was glued to the weather channel for the next 36 hours, napping on the couch so I would not miss a report. It was just too horrible to imagine. I feared the worst. (My motto, expect the worst and hope for the best). As the day progressed, my anxiety increased. It was bad, I knew it.

I had volunteered to baby-sit Liz's friend's sick four month old baby girl, so fortunately I was distracted on Tuesday, August 30. CNN and the baby kept me busy until mid morning and finally the call. It was Gene's office in Washington. They had just heard from Gene and the family was safe. Dean's home had roof damage, but they were ok. The Bay houses were not. Neither made it. Our family home and Gene's home were gone. My old Waveland home, built to be indestructible, was also gone.

My worst fear became a reality. As with most traumatic times in my life, I have post trauma breakdowns and this was another of those times. The baby began crying, and I walked and rocked in a daze. I called Bob and told him the news, then Sue. Gone. So many memories gone, but thank God the family had made it. I did think of Mom and was so glad she didn't have to live through that. But, I know she could have, and I know we all can too.

The rest is history. On August 29, 2005, our Coast experienced the worst national disaster in United States history. Hurricane Katrina's 125 mile-per-hour winds and 34-foot storm surge put 95% of the Bay-Waveland area under water. The water surged inland seven miles, submerging homes, businesses and even the I-10 interstate highway. The connection to the rest of the coast, our two-mile long Bay Bridge along highway 90 was dismembered. Our centuries old community, with it's antebellum mansions along Beach Boulevard, and the artists' galleries in the town center were either leveled or left in piles of rubble. There were 231 fatalities in the three South Mississippi counties and around 67 people still missing. Our local paper, the Sun Herald, reported that 65,380 homes were destroyed and that the Gulf Coast had sustained an estimated $125 billion dollars in damages. So much lost, yet much more remembered.

I am so proud of my brothers and their families. Dean and Marilene had six families living with them through the storm and in the following weeks. Gene and his teenage son, Gary, were so active in search and rescue. One can't even imagine the devastation and carnage they encountered.

My second trip to the Bay was in February 2006, six months after the storm. Everything was still so sad. Not much had changed. There are three families now living on the farm. Daily struggles with the insurance companies, and enormous amounts of paperwork. The planning and waiting are emotionally and physically draining. Yet, as always, there is so much hope, love and a little sprinkle of fun.

Love between the three families (Dean's, Gene's, and Rosemary) has blended them beautifully into one. Yes, they were close before, but now it is different. Although successful career men and women, they spend every waking hour clearing the property and struggling to rebuild, just like everyone else in town. They support each other, and that love and support radiates throughout the farm.

We always have hope. Mom would be so proud. Gene and Margaret work tirelessly to keep our cause visible nationally and in fundraising for rebuilding.

Did I forget the fun? Oh, no way. My trip coincided with our Mardi Gras celebration. After so much stress, frustration and sadness, this town desperately needed a party.

Upon hearing that my brother Gene was to be the Grand Marshall for the Nereids parade, I imposed upon my sister in Baton Rouge, and Di and Michael went with me for the weekend. We met the family and had a few wonderful hours, screaming, yelling and catching beads. I realized I had not been to a parade since I left Waveland, 25 years ago, and I vowed not to miss another one.

Later we drove by my old home on the beach in Waveland. Almost gone…yet so many memories. I stood on the steps where I have a photo of myself with a suitcase in my hand, going to the Slidell hospital to have Charlotte. Di took this picture of me then. Now, only the slab and steps remain. Tears spilled over my cheeks as I recalled that clear October day 27 years ago, and remembered all the love and hard work we put into that place for three years. But it is the view I will always remember, blue sky, glistening water gently breaking on the seawall, and a few seagulls flying effortlessly overhead.

Back on the farm, the boys boiled crabs for the family and after a wonderful meal we sat together to watch CNN's Kathleen Koch's documentary *Saving my town: Bay St. Louis, Mississippi.* Back to reality, Katrina constantly haunts them.

We are now in the beginning of the next hurricane season, but we are also 75 days away from the next party! There will be another family wedding to take place in Bay St. Louis in August. Believe it or not, Our Lady of the Gulf Church on the beach is ready as well as the Parish hall. One way or another, the best band on the Coast has been secured and "The good times will roll." Now we have something to look forward to.

As with so many other areas of my life, the Coast and New Orleans are almost gone…but they too will survive and not be forgotten. We are all survivors and I have a little more peace now that I know my new guardian angel is watching out for us. Thanks, Momsy, for the strong foundation you set for our family, and especially for all the lessons you taught me. Without your love and support, I never could have made it through all these hurricanes. I am truly blessed.

Larry's Laws for the Loveless

Be Patient.

Divorces usually take at least a year.

Good things take time!

Be Calm.

You (and the children) will adjust.

Time does heal all wounds, and all wounds do heal.

Expect the Worst.

Keep in mind that in the legal system, NOTHING is engraved in stone! (The court date, the deposition, the legal fees…)

Delays are likely to occur NUMEROUS times.

Hang in There.

There is life after divorce.

With every end there is a new beginning.

Go For It!

Licking the Lumpectomy: A Therapist's Tips for Treating the Tittie

Week one: Hospital Admission and Surgery

Read the Fine Print!

Don't sign the release form unless you and the surgeon agree to what will still be there when you wake up! A miscommunication here could really be devastating.

Talk to the anesthesiologist.

Although the cheap version of the anesthesia works OK on 99% of the population, give yourself a break and ask for the "high dollar" stuff! Nausea is the pits and this is not where you are thinking about a good dollar value. You have probably met the deductible on you insurance, so go for the Jose Cuervo Gold. It is worth it!

Waking Up

You did wake up!
But don't get too clear headed. You usually do have pain, so take the pain medicine as often as possible. It works great. Sorry, this expensive hotel does not serve wine or margaritas, so get the next best medicine without the hangover!

Going Home

Oh God, I'm radioactive! No, Scottie will not beam you up, so enjoy the peace and quiet and snooze. No visitors today, but not to worry, your husband can tape Oprah for you, and you can catch it tomorrow.

Next day, you lost two pounds! Aren't these resorts just great! Now you and your spouse can pretend you're on the set of ER twice a day. Get those bandages ready for the dressing changes, and don't forget the Vitamin E cream for the scar (when healed of course).

Empty the drain bag daily, and be thankful it doesn't show you what's in your stomach. It too, is temporary, so hide the darn thing under your shirt. (Do not pin it to your pants or you'll be in trouble when you need to go potty.)

Week Two

Your New Wardrobe

Forget about all that Victoria Secret stuff for the next two months. You are now into exercise wear. Close your eyes and imagine you are back at Wimbledon, and you are getting ready to play tennis not watch it. Don that sports bra and go. Be sure to have a wide variety of colors on hand to mix and match with your slacks. When you get bummed, just think about all the money you saved on dry cleaning, and how much fun you're going to have spending it later!

Exercises

Now that you are "snug as a bug in a rug" prepare for those overheads. The best place to begin this is in the shower. Let the warm water run over your shoulder, lean over and gently start making circles with your arm. Just loosen it up by making circles in both directions, forward and backwards, and out to the side. Then try reaching toward the shower head. If the pressure from the water is too painful, turn around and let the water hit the back of your shoulder. Keep reaching until you feel a little pull in your chest, and gradually try to lift it higher everyday. Keep working it in the shower and try to bring your arm out to the side, up and over the head to reach the other shoulder. (Yes, this is possible!)

Don't despair, there should be plenty of Vicodin left so don't be a martyr. As one doctor told me, "You do not get extra points for suffering!"

Radiation

Welcome to the Oncology Center. (You just found out what Oncology means). After the initial shock wears off, just keep telling yourself that all of those sick looking old people are Not like you. You are younger, stronger, and a fighter. You have a lot to live for and you are thankful that it is you that has cancer rather than your, mother, sister, or sister in law. One out of eight women we know have it, right? (lucky us). Well, we will make it.

Another pile of papers is given for you to sort through. In a nutshell this is what they say: No deodorant on the affected side, another new experience, sweating on one side only! You must avoid the sun like the plague. Cornstarch may be used under the effected arm for the next 6 ½ weeks. 5 ½ weeks of the regular radiation and then THE BOOST! The boost is the last Zap directed right to the cancer site. Oh, by the way, you may feel a little tired as the weeks progress and the cumulative effect kicks in along with a little itching. Now these are Real Hot Tips!

The real skinny on this is: the actual process of receiving the radiation treatment is a piece of cake. Your surgeon placed little clips inside you to point directly to the cancer site (don't worry about these, you can't move them around while you are massaging the scar). Now the oncologist will know where to aim those big, scary machines. Close your eyes and counts to 60 slowly, one side down, then they move the machine toward the other X spot, and Kazaam! Its over.

Dealing with the visual reminders of your cancer was the biggest nightmare. Not the scarlet letter, but the Aqua Box! Although this young generation thinks tattoos are cool, I personally had a hard time with my new "body art"

This is a big hurdle to jump. I since found out that other places, like the University of Michigan and Sloan Kettering, use a very small mole size tattoo for their markings, but here in Texas it's "not the MD Anderson way". Please. Doctors can be so inflexible!

If you don't need the support of the sports bra anymore, head to Target for some cheap cotton camisoles. The black ink will still get on your camisole, but think of the fun you'll have burning it when your done! You may also start to get sore from the Zapping, so get the Aloe Vera gel and rub it around the area. They should give you some aqua something gel and that is only for the ninny! That's the reason the tube is so small.

Advil had been recommended to me for the pain. However, since anti-inflammatory drugs have been scratched from my list of acceptable meds, I have relied on Margaritas, Vodka, or Tylenol (not all together,) as a last resort to take the edge off. When the itching has you patting your chest all day like Tarzan, its time for

Benadryl. Hopefully, you won't have to operate any heavy machinery, for drowsiness is a side affect.

When sleeping becomes a problem, and the above remedies are not cutting it, they have a pill for that too. Thorazine. It is magic. You are off to La La land in no time and wake up ready to play.

Later Weeks

Mental Health Check

But you look great! That expensive French makeup you bought is finally paying off. Like Nana always said, "a little powder, a little paint makes you look like what you ain't!" Amen. You need to use it when you just stay home. We know that although you are making it through the day, you are still suffering inside.

From the moment you heard the news, your life has probably been a nightmare. You can't forget about it even for a few minutes. It always seems to haunt you. Just when you think you are OK, some little thing your husband does or the kids do, just sets you off and you go ballistic. You are back in the crying jag, for now crying seems like a way of life rather than an emotion. You're sure you are the ugliest creature on the earth, you feel like hell, and nobody understands. Your husband and kids have been great but this is beginning to take its toll on them too. Your radiation techs have come around and are now used to your mood swings, but you only see them a few minutes a day.

Then all of a sudden you have a new friend. She comes for treatment right after you and she actually smiled at you. Happiness is someone who has been there and understands. Your "wine and whine" friend.

For the first time in weeks, you feel like you just might make it. This person is a great listener, and non-judgmental. To her, you are not whining or complaining, you are sharing your feelings. A support group without the group!

Be sure and find a friend or support group, it is better than all the reading material in the world. There is nothing like a warm body to listen to and hug with when you need it. And you do need it! Something good just might come out of this. Like Dad said "things do work out for the best".

Now go on that celebration trip, you made it! Have a great time, for now you are out of the umbrella of the "Big C." Eat, drink and be merry for tomorrow we won't die! We made it through with the insurance policy, remember? Life can, and will only get better. Let's go for it!

978-0-595-39156-1
0-595-39156-7

www.ingramcontent.com/pod-product-compliance
Lightning Source LLC
Chambersburg PA
CBHW051431280526
45785CB00003B/1246